Newborn Life Su

CW01024704

4th Edition February 2016

Reprinted in September 2016

978-1-903812-33-4

Editors

Jonathan Wyllie
Sean Ainsworth
Robert Tinnion
Sue Hampshire

Contributors

This Newborn Life Support (NLS) manual is written by the Resuscitation Council (UK) NLS Subcommittee and forms part of the resources for the Resuscitation Council (UK) NLS course, which is delivered in accredited course centres throughout the UK. Members of the Subcommittee:

Jonathan Wyllie
Sean Ainsworth
Alison Bedford-Russell
Andy Coleman
Rowan Davies
Sue Hampshire

Hilary Lumsden
John Madar
Stephanie Michaelides
Sarah Mitchell
Vix Monnelly
Niall Pearcey

Eleri Pritchard
Mark Sedge
Rachel Tennant
Rob Tinnion
Vivienne van Someren

Colour plates reproduced with permission of the Northern Neonatal Network who retain copyright.

Environmental friendly paper has been used. 15% recycled, elemental chlorine free fibre sourced from well managed forests.

Published by © Resuscitation Council (UK) 2016
5th Floor, Tavistock House North, Tavistock Square, London WC1H 9HR
Tel: 020 7388 4678 Fax: 020 7383 0773 email: enquiries@resus.org.uk website: www.resus.org.uk

Design & Print: TT Litho Printers Limited
Units 3 & 5 Northpoint, Enterprise Close, Medway City Estate, Rochester, Kent ME2 4LX
Tel: 01634 845397 Email: admin@ttlitho.co.uk Website: http://www.ttlitho.co.uk

Contents

Acknowledgements

This text started life in the UK in 1980 as a small booklet written to help midwives, nurses and doctors faced, for the first time, with a responsibility for the care of babies at birth. Early editions were written by Dr Edmund Hey who, as a physiologist working with Professor Kenneth Cross in the 1960s, was involved in much of the original research into the physiology of neonatal asphyxia and temperature control. They were written to complement a regional theoretical and practical course in newborn resuscitation in the Northern Health Region of the United Kingdom. The booklet remained a locally written text, though with considerable national and a small international distribution, through a number of editions published by the Northern Neonatal Network. The fifth and final edition appeared in 1996. The working group is grateful to the Network for permission to reproduce their physiological diagrams. Dr Hey retired from his post as consultant neonatologist at the Princess Mary Maternity Hospital in Newcastle upon Tyne in 1994 and died in 2009.

When the Resuscitation Council (UK) set up a working group to develop the Newborn Life Support course Dr Sam Richmond, a long-time colleague and collaborator of Dr Hey, was appointed as chair. He was the editor of the first three versions of the NLS manual and closely involved in all aspects of the course and materials. Even after stepping down as chair, he remained involved as a member of the working group until shortly before his death in March 2013 and it is impossible to overestimate the loss of his giant intellect and encyclopaedic knowledge of the literature. He was also a chair of the NLS international Courses Committee of the European Resuscitation Council (ERC) and past co-chair of the neonatal task force of the International Liaison Committee on Resuscitation (ILCOR), evaluating evidence and writing guidelines from 2005 to 2010. He was made a Fellow of the ERC and an Honorary Member of the Resuscitation Council UK in recognition of his contributions to resuscitation knowledge and training. The working group would all want to acknowledge his lasting contribution upon which this manual is built.

We also would like to acknowledge the inspiration and constructive challenges afforded by regular meetings and conversations with Professors Jeffrey Perlman, John Kattwinkel, Myra Wyckoff and all the members of the neonatal section of the International Liaison Committee on Resuscitation (ILCOR) over the past 15 years. Any reader interested in exploring the evidence behind the various recommendations made in this and other texts on the topic of neonatal resuscitation are urged to access the evidence evaluations carried out in 2010 and 2015. There are hyperlinks in these documents to the relevant worksheets.

The URL is:

2015 http://www.resuscitationjournal.com/article/S0300-9572(15)00366-4/pdf

2010 http://circ.ahajournals.org/content/122/16_suppl_2/S516.full

Finally we would like to acknowledge the input, discussions and innovations in approach brought about by the interaction with the working group which developed the Advanced Resuscitation of the Newborn Infant course, especially the editors Drs Joe Fawke and Jonathan Cusack and also Dr Fiona Wood for developments in teaching facemask ventilation.

The Newborn Life Support course

Aims of the NLS course

Having read the manual and completed a Newborn Life Support course you should:

1. **Understand the physiological processes underlying apnoea, bradycardia and poor condition at birth after a hypoxic insult.**

2. **Be able to anticipate which babies who may have problems, assess a baby at birth and recognise those who require additional help.**

3. **Be able to describe and follow the principles of a standardised approach to resuscitation of babies in need of assistance at birth, emphasising the overriding importance of airway management and lung inflation, and the limited role for chest compressions and drugs.**

4. **Have had practical experience in appropriate handling of the equipment used in newborn resuscitation.**

5. **Have learnt core skills in the management of the newborn airway including strategies to help in situations where the initial attempt at lung inflation is unsuccessful.**

6. **Have been taught, performed and, in respect of the management of Airway and Breathing, been assessed on the following skills on manikins:**

    -   **Airway management and lung inflation and aeration**

    -   **Direct laryngoscopic inspection of the oropharynx**

    -   **Chest compressions**

    -   **Umbilical venous access.**

7. **Have practiced and received constructive feedback about the immediate management of newborn emergencies in simulations with an appreciation of the importance of communication and teamwork.**

8. **Have demonstrated, in a test simulation using manikins, the core skills of airway management of a newborn infant and subsequent, structured, management steps if initial attempts are unsuccessful.**

9. **Have developed a framework for succinct recording and effective communication of important details of the baby's condition at birth and the response to resuscitation.**

10. **Have practised the skills and developed an approach to newborn resuscitation during the first 10–20 minutes after birth as a basis to build upon with further mentored clinical training, which will permit achievement of clinical competence.**

The Newborn Life Support (NLS) course has been developed, under the auspices of the Resuscitation Council (UK), to provide clear practical instruction in resuscitation of babies at birth. It is designed for all health workers, regardless of their discipline or status, who may be called upon to resuscitate a newborn baby. The course is supported by the Royal College of Midwives, the British Association of Perinatal Medicine and the Royal College of Paediatrics and Child Health.

Why babies at birth are different and which need resuscitation

Contents

- **The physiological and anatomical differences between newborn babies and other age groups and the impact of these on resuscitation**
- **Defining "resuscitation" and some of the essential differences in the approach required when dealing with babies at birth**
- **How many babies may need intervention at birth from a practitioner trained in newborn resuscitation**
- **How many deliveries may require the presence of a practitioner trained in newborn resuscitation in anticipation of that need**

Learning outcomes

To enable you to:

- **Understand what is different about babies at birth**
- **Consider how these differences affect the approach to resuscitation**
- **Describe the difference between "resuscitation" and "assisted transition" (or stabilisation)**
- **Consider the frequency of newborn resuscitation**

Why babies at birth are different

Introduction

Humans require immediate, life-saving assistance when breathing is interrupted, the circulation fails, or both. The immediate interventions that can be performed to aid recovery from this situation are generally termed "resuscitation". Newborn babies are frequently reported as needing "resuscitation" after birth. However there are a number of differences between babies at birth and later on in life.

Babies at birth are not only smaller than adults and older children but are also physiologically different, and may need resuscitation for different reasons. A different approach to the resuscitation of a newborn baby is therefore necessary from that adopted with a collapsed child or adult.

Adults

In adults, collapse requiring resuscitation is usually due to a cardiac event, most commonly myocardial infarction, pulseless arrhythmia, or both. Breathing stops because oxygen is no longer being delivered to the respiratory centre in the brainstem. The resuscitator therefore has to reproduce the action of both the heart and the lungs in the hope of preserving flow of adequately oxygenated blood to the heart and brain. This is done using chest compressions and lung ventilation usually referred to as cardiopulmonary resuscitation (CPR). The problem with the heart has to be diagnosed and treated usually requiring an ECG (or cardiac monitor), defibrillator, and occasionally, drugs. Throughout the time taken to do this, oxygen supply to the brain must be maintained using CPR to minimise subsequent neurological damage.

Children

In children, collapse requiring resuscitation is usually respiratory in aetiology, which may lead to myocardial compromise and cardiac arrest. However the underlying pathologies are many and varied.

Babies

Being delivered through the birth canal is a hypoxic experience for the fetus because respiratory exchange via the placenta is interrupted for the 50–75 s duration of the average contraction. Though most babies tolerate this well, some do not and these few may require help to establish normal breathing at delivery. Thus, in newborn babies the problem is almost always one requiring primarily respiratory support.

The heart of the newborn baby can continue functioning for 20 minutes or more despite anoxia. The newborn baby at term has evolved to undertake the strenuous passage through the birth canal and the brain of these babies can withstand lack of oxygen for much longer than an adult brain. During prolonged anoxia, however, the neural mechanisms driving attempts at normal breathing and the 'reserve' spinal reflex of anoxic gasping will cease to function if they are unsuccessful in drawing air into the lungs (Chapter 4).

To resuscitate a newborn baby it is sufficient, in most cases, to aerate the lungs. The newborn lung is fluid-filled at birth, which makes the technique of initial lung aeration different. Whilst the fluid starts to be reabsorbed with the onset of labour, vaginally delivered babies at term still have about 70 mL of lung fluid to be absorbed. Those born by section prior to the onset of labour may have more fluid to clear.

In most cases of newborn 'resuscitation' the circulation is usually still functioning and, following 'aeration' or 'inflation' of the lungs, can then direct oxygenated blood back to the heart from the lungs, leading to recovery. In rare instances the heart may need a brief period of chest compressions to achieve the same movement of oxygenated blood before the circulation is restored. The significant primary rhythm problems seen in adults do not occur, therefore the devices needed to deal with these cardiac arrhythmias that dominate adult resuscitation are unnecessary and even drugs are rarely needed.

Babies get cold easily

Babies are small and have a high surface-area-to-weight ratio. They are also born wet. These factors mean that babies can lose heat rapidly after birth, especially if requiring resuscitation. Special measures are required to maintain the temperature in the normal range of 36.5°C to 37.5°C because both hypothermia and hyperthermia are associated with increased mortality and morbidity at all gestations.

Resuscitation, or "assisted transition"?

In adult medicine the term "resuscitation" is usually used to describe the urgent application of ventilation, chest compression, and often defibrillation, to an apparently lifeless adult.

Many discussions in the paediatric literature start with the unreferenced assertion that "resuscitation" of the baby is necessary following 6 to 10% of all births. In the few studies that have examined this critically the need to apply both ventilation and chest compression to an apparently lifeless baby at birth is a rare event, occurring in about 1 in 2000 deliveries in countries with highly developed health care. [1] Approximately 85% of babies born at term will initiate spontaneous respirations within 10 to 30 s of birth; an additional 10 % will respond during drying and stimulation, and approximately 3% will initiate respirations following positive pressure ventilation. [2-4]

In the context of newborn babies it is clear that the term "resuscitation" is often used somewhat loosely. Some babies are clearly severely unwell at delivery and are, unarguably, in need of urgent attention to restore vital functions and this might legitimately be described as 'resuscitation'. However, this is not the usual experience of an attendant called to help a baby at delivery. In most cases, what is required is 'stabilisation' to assist the transition from placental to pulmonary respiration. [5] This is particularly true of the preterm infant where there is not usually a hypoxic insult.

How big is the problem?

Given that neonatal resuscitation is rarely defined in any detail, the frequency it is actually needed is difficult to determine. Furthermore, the fact that a baby received resuscitative measures at birth does not mean that the baby required such measures to ensure survival.

A study at one hospital showed a fall in intubation rate from 7% to 1.5% following a change in policy, which had resulted in fewer deliveries being attended by a paediatrician. One interpretation of this might be that a major 'risk factor' for intubation at birth was the presence of a paediatrician. [6] Information from Scottish hospitals in the 1980s showed that between 8–12% of babies born at a major hospital in Edinburgh received tracheal intubation at birth, whereas this occurred in only 1.5–2% of those born at a comparable hospital in Aberdeen. [7] The latter data correlate well with that from the 1990s in the north of England. [8]

Airway and breathing

Perhaps the best information available on the need for resuscitation rather than its use comes from a study in Sweden. [9] All 97,648 births in that country over a one year period were studied. A standard approach was taught in Sweden that advocated mask inflation initially with progress to intubation only if mask inflation was not successful. Amongst babies weighing 2.5 kg or more, only about 10 babies per 1000 received mask inflation or intubation. Of these babies 8 per 1000 responded to mask inflation and only 2 per 1000 seemed to require intubation at birth. [9] This conclusion is supported by a much smaller UK study involving about 18,000 deliveries at one hospital over 4 years which found that only 4 babies per 1000 over 37 weeks gestation were intubated in the last year of the study. [10] Although overall perinatal mortality figures are lower in Scandinavia than the UK, the birthweight-specific perinatal mortality rates of the two populations are very similar. [11]

The equipment available for mask inflation 40 years ago was less effective than it is today because it was not designed for positive pressure ventilation. As a result lack of confidence in this method was then widespread, which probably explains the high intubation rates at that time. When masks specifically designed for positive pressure ventilation were introduced in the mid-1980s [12] it was not surprising that it took a little time for this scepticism to disappear. These new masks, when used correctly, are able to aerate the lungs effectively and the perceived 'need' for intubation at delivery in the UK has fallen considerably in the past 20 years.

Chest compressions and drugs

In adult resuscitation the most effective intervention is usually defibrillation with chest compressions being used to maintain a circulation to the brain and heart until such time as a defibrillator can be applied.

In babies, the crucial intervention is to aerate and then ventilate the lungs. Chest compression is needed in a very few cases and then only to assist the heart in delivering oxygenated blood to the coronary arteries and the heart muscle. The cartilaginous rib cage of the newborn and the larger size of the heart relative to the chest make chest compression much easier as well as more efficient.

An American study over two years found only 39 (0.12%) of 30,839 infants were administered chest compressions and/or adrenaline (epinephrine) as part of cardiopulmonary resuscitation in the delivery room. Of these 15 were term infants and 24 were premature.[13] In the context of newborn babies it is clear that the term 'resuscitation' is often used somewhat loosely and that 'resuscitation' beyond maintenance of normal temperature and management of airway and breathing is, therefore, a rare occurrence in newborn babies.

Which deliveries should be attended by a practitioner trained in newborn resuscitation?

Many labour ward policies suggest the need for a practitioner trained in newborn resuscitation to attend a delivery is determined by the mode of delivery. A typical policy might demand attendance at all sections, all breech deliveries, all multiple deliveries, all instrumental deliveries, all preterm deliveries, all deliveries where monitoring (e.g. with cardiotocograph) suggests fetal compromise and all meconium staining. Such a policy would involve attending more than 30% of deliveries and would not eliminate the need for urgent calls to resuscitate babies found to be unexpectedly unresponsive at birth.[14] A more logical approach would be to relate the need to attend a delivery to the anticipated condition of the baby.

One study reported the efforts of paediatricians to reduce an attendance rate of 39% of deliveries to 25%. [6] Despite attending 39% of deliveries there were 20 further deliveries (1.5% of deliveries) where help was apparently required but had not been expected and this proportion neither increased nor decreased when new policies were introduced.

Whatever guidelines are used to determine the presence of a practitioner trained in newborn resuscitation some babies will be born who unexpectedly require resuscitation. It is, therefore, very important that everyone who takes on the responsibility of delivering babies should be trained in resuscitation at birth.

Summary learning

- **Babies are small and wet at birth and must be kept warm. Those that need resuscitation at birth have a respiratory problem. Once air enters the lungs, the heart usually responds. It follows that after making sure a baby is kept warm, the most important skill to learn is that of effective airway management and successful lung aeration.**

- **Most babies do not need resuscitation and breathe within 10–30 s of birth or after drying.**

- **Of the 5% of babies who receive resuscitative intervention, most respond after effective aeration of the lungs.**

- **Most preterm infants merely require stabilisation to achieve transition not resuscitation.**

My key take-home messages from this chapter

NLS

General care at birth

Contents

- **Initial actions at birth**
- **Maintaining normothermia (temperature between 36.5°C and 37.5°C)**
- **Assessment of the newly born baby**
- **Care of the baby who does not need help; parents, feeding, examination, washing**

Learning outcomes

To enable you to:

- **Describe the immediate management of newborn babies, including the majority who do not require any assistance with the transition to the extra-uterine environment**
- **Understand how to assess babies in the first minutes after birth to decide whether they need intervention or normal postnatal care**

Introduction

Most mature babies will breathe or cry within 90 s of birth, some others need a little assistance and very few need resuscitation, even after an operative delivery. However, every newborn baby should be individually assessed at birth.

It is not necessary to spend time trying to remove small amounts of liquor from the mouth and nose because the average 3 kg baby will clear more than 100 mL of fluid from the lungs and trachea quite unaided in a matter of minutes. [15, 16] They do not need to be held head down, given oxygen or subjected to vigorous suction but should be dried and wrapped in dry towels to minimise heat loss.

Pause to assess the baby

In utero the baby respires via the placenta. After birth this function is taken over by the lungs. Following *normal* birth a *gradual* transition from one method of respiration to the other occurs. This can take a few minutes to complete, though in most instances it happens very quickly. While this is happening redistribution of blood between the placenta and the baby is also occurring. If the placenta is still attached to the uterine wall, and if the baby appears well, then there is no need to interrupt this process.

It is important to assess the baby (see below) because in those babies not in need of resuscitation it is recommended that the cord should not be clamped for *at least* one minute after the baby emerges. [17, 18] In stable babies it is logical to clamp the cord after respirations have become established but only if the baby is kept warm. To prevent heat loss the baby can be wrapped, and if placed skin to skin, should also be covered, during this interval. Very early clamping may cause hypovolaemia. [19, 20] For a more detailed discussion of the timing of cord clamping see Appendix 1.

Warmth

Keeping the baby warm is essential. Because of their small size and relatively large surface area babies can get cold very quickly. The human fetus has a higher temperature (approximately 0.5°C) than its mother [21] and can become very cold very quickly after birth without active management; one baby, born by an unattended delivery at home, was reported to have a core temperature of 18°C when admitted to hospital 40 min after delivery. [22] Even in a delivery room, if left naked and wet, the baby's temperature can fall to 33°C within 5 min. [23] Ideally the baby should be born into an environment that is warm enough to allow the baby to maintain a body temperature within the normal range without effort. Babies subjected to cold stress in the period immediately after births have a lower oxygen tension [24] and an increased metabolic acidosis. [25] There is evidence in animals that hypoxia, acidosis and hypothermia all tend to inhibit surfactant production. [26]

The admission temperature of newly born infants is a strong predictor of mortality and morbidity at all gestations [27, 28] and should be recorded as a predictor of outcome as well as a quality indicator. [17, 18] Hypothermia after birth continues to be a worldwide problem in all settings. [27-31] It is associated with increased mortality and morbidity especially in small and preterm babies. For every 1°C below 36.5°C the risk of mortality increases by up to 28%. [32, 33] The temperature of all newly born infants who are not being considered for therapeutic hypothermia should be maintained between 36.5°C and 37.5°C after birth through admission and stabilization.

Methods of heat loss

Heat loss occurs by four different routes: evaporation, convection, conduction and radiation. When the skin is wet with amniotic fluid, moisture quickly evaporates from the skin's surface taking a large amount of heat with it as latent heat of evaporation. Draughts of air moving past the baby encourage this and also cause loss of heat by convection. Placing the baby on a cold surface such as cool mattresses or towels will risk heat loss by conduction. Finally the baby may lose heat by radiation from uncovered skin surfaces direct to cooler surfaces. In the newborn baby most heat is lost by evaporation and convection.

Preventing heat loss

There are several simple and effective ways by which heat loss can be kept to a minimum:

- Dry the baby and wrap in a pre-warmed towel to prevent evaporative heat loss. [34]

- Keep the delivery area draught free by keeping doors and windows shut wherever possible, to reduce heat loss by convection. [35, 36]

- Maintain the environmental temperature within the range 23–25°C. [36-38]

- Place the baby skin-to-skin and cover. [39-45]

- If the baby needs attention place the baby on a warm mattress under a radiant heater to reduce heat loss by radiation and conduction.

It is likely that a combination of methods will be required to maintain the temperature in babies who require help (chapter 8).

Initial assessment

Allow the baby a minute or two to adjust before clamping and cutting the cord as above. During this time keep the baby warm and assess:

**Colour
Tone
Breathing
Heart Rate**

The items are listed in this order because this is the order in which this information becomes available. Colour can be assessed as soon as you see the baby, tone can be appreciated as soon as you see and touch the baby, breathing can be noted almost as quickly but detection of heart rate requires a little more time. Reassess heart rate and breathing regularly during any subsequent resuscitation, as these are the first to change and can be used to guide your actions.

Colour

Look at the colour of the trunk, lips and tongue. Most babies appear blue at first and can remain so for several minutes after birth; in itself this does not mean the baby requires assistance. Other elements of the assessment are needed to fully guide any interventions.

Tone

Note whether the baby is well flexed with good tone or floppy like a rag doll.

Breathing

Look at the rate and pattern of respiration. Most babies start breathing regularly within 30 s of birth. In one national UK study over 75% of surviving babies established regular breathing by 60 s. However around 20% of otherwise normal babies took between 60–180 s to start breathing regularly. [46] Gasping respirations are usually a sign that the baby will need help.

Heart rate

Listen for the heart rate with a stethoscope or feel for a pulse at the base of the umbilical cord. In an apnoeic baby the slow pulsation of the ventricles can often be seen lifting the chest wall. Even in a healthy baby the cord does not always pulsate, nor does the rate of cord pulsation always reflect the true pulse rate. If you feel a normal heart rate of over 100 beats min^{-1} in the cord it suggests all is well. However, if you feel a slow heart rate or no pulse at all this may not reflect the true heart rate. [47] Check with a stethoscope or a pulse oximeter.

Interpretation

A baby who is initially blue but breathing regularly, with a fast heart rate, and who has good tone needs no further intervention (other than to maintain its temperature) and may be given to the mother. A further assessment should be made of the colour to check this is continuing to improve but if the baby is breathing regularly this need not involve anything more than a quick visual check.

A baby who is not breathing adequately, who has a slow heart rate or one who is blue-white or floppy should be dried and covered and, if the situation allows, placed under a radiant heat source, so that further actions may then be taken.

CALL FOR HELP IF YOU FEEL YOU NEED IT

Parents

At delivery, do not take the baby away from the mother unless this is clearly necessary. Both parents may want to hold and examine their baby and, if the baby appears well, they should be encouraged to do so once the baby has been dried, and assuming the delivery area is warm and draught free. This is also a very good time to initiate breast feeding. Mature babies are at very little risk of becoming cold while they remain in the warmth of their mother's arms, even if unclothed (skin-to-skin), as long as the mother and baby are protected from draughts by a blanket and the environment is warm (Figure 3.1). [34, 48] Respect the family's need for peace and privacy but ensure that the airway of these babies is not compromised. [49-51]

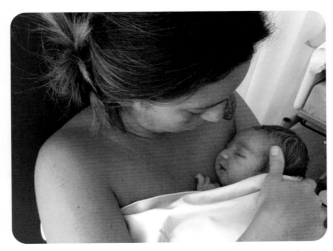

Figure 3.1 Baby skin-to-skin, covered, in supported position but without head covering.

Early feeding

All babies experience a fall in blood glucose in the first few hours after birth. The lowest point of this fall can reach levels of 1–2 mmol L^{-1}. [52] This level in adults would cause unconsciousness or even fitting but does not do so in appropriately grown term newborn babies because alternative fuels for the brain are usually easily available in the form of lactate and ketones. Lactate is relatively high at birth and falls in the first few hours, thus providing alternative brain fuel while blood glucose production from glycogen is initiated. [53] Within a few hours of birth most babies start to produce ketones which can also be used as brain fuel and which will be available for the first 72 h or so while breast feeding becomes established. [53]

Preterm babies (less than 37 weeks) and babies who are wasted or small for gestational age are less able to produce this protective ketogenic response. [54] Infants of insulin-dependent diabetic mothers may have an apparently higher requirement for glucose. [55] Some maternal medications may also impair a baby's ability to maintain blood sugar. [56] Babies who get cold, and thus have to use energy to try to maintain their body temperature, will use up their fuel reserves more rapidly. There is no need to wash the baby at birth. Doing so makes the baby very cold unnecessarily. [34]

Examination

The baby should be briefly examined shortly after birth and in the presence of the parents. This examination should check for any signs of cardio-respiratory distress, congenital anomalies or injuries that may have occurred during the birthing process. The baby must be kept warm during this process and all findings should be recorded in the baby notes. A more detailed examination will take place later.

Summary learning

- **An initial assessment of the baby's condition can be made quickly after birth.**

- **Allow time for placental transfusion if immediate resuscitation is not required.**

- **The importance of drying and covering the baby to prevent heat loss cannot be over emphasised.**

- **Do not take the baby away from the parents unless it is clearly necessary.**

My key take-home messages from this chapter

Physiology of transition at birth and perinatal hypoxia

Contents

- **The normal physiology of birth and the potential effect of cord clamping**
- **The historical approaches to resuscitation and the findings of the animal research on which the modern approach to resuscitation at birth is based**
- **The response of the fetus to acute hypoxia at birth and the naturally occurring protective mechanisms**
- **How the physiological data allows a logical approach to supporting transition at birth and resuscitation, when needed, to be developed**

Learning outcomes

To enable you to:

- **Understand the normal physiology of transition at birth**
- **Describe the pathophysiology of acute perinatal hypoxia**

Introduction to the terminology used

Many of the terms used in describing the events during the transition to air breathing carry medico-legal as well as pathophysiological implications. Unfortunately the terms have been used quite interchangeably and somewhat loosely in the past. The following is a list of terms that may be found in texts and papers on the subject:

Acidaemia	Increased concentration of hydrogen ions in blood
Acidosis	Increased concentration of hydrogen ions in any tissue. A respiratory acidosis arises when there is an accumulation of carbon dioxide (which is converted into carbonic acid). A metabolic acidosis arises when there is an accumulation of acids that arise from the body's metabolism (such as lactic acid, which is produced as a by-product of anaerobic metabolism, or any one of a number of organic acids that accumulate in inherited metabolic conditions). A mixed acidosis has both respiratory and other components
Anoxia	Lack of oxygen in any tissue
Asphyxia	A condition in which an extreme decrease in the concentration of oxygen in the body leads to loss of consciousness or death
	The term is now obsolete (and therefore best avoided), having been replaced in the mid-twentieth century by the more specific terms anoxia, hypoxia, hypoxaemia and hypercapnia
Hypercapnia (also hypercarbia)	Abnormally high levels of carbon dioxide in the blood
Hypoxaemia	Decreased oxygen content of blood
Hypoxia	Decreased level of oxygen in any tissue

Birth physiology and transition

Birth represents a significant physiological challenge for a fetus in changing from a liquid-filled *in utero* environment to independent life in air. [57, 58] Although most babies undergo this change without difficulty, some infants, particularly those born prematurely, require assistance most commonly in the form of respiratory support. [57] During fetal life, the lungs are liquid-filled and gas exchange occurs across the placenta. [59, 60] Following cessation of placental function the lungs must take over this role. To achieve this, the alveoli must be aerated and blood flow through the lungs must increase significantly. [58, 61] Aeration of the lungs triggers a decrease in pulmonary vascular resistance and an increase in pulmonary blood flow. Whilst aeration is the primary driver for the increase in pulmonary blood flow the exact mechanisms governing this event remain unclear. [62] Increased oxygenation, mediated by nitric oxide release, [62] is one component of the response, but mechanisms independent of oxygen are also involved. [63, 64]

During normal labour, recurrent uterine contraction interferes with placental gas exchange resulting in a degree of fetal hypoxia. [65] The process of labour stimulates production of adrenaline by the fetus [66] and thyrotropin releasing hormone by the mother. [67] This encourages the cells responsible for secreting lung fluid in the fetus to cease production and to begin to absorb fluid from the alveolar spaces, preparing the lungs for air breathing.

At birth the loss of umbilical blood flow may significantly reduce venous return for both ventricles if pulmonary blood flow does not simultaneously increase. [68, 69] Observational studies of heart rate at birth in normal healthy infants show a reduction in heart rates immediately after birth increasing within a few minutes [70], a finding first published more than 50 years ago by Brady and James [71] with immediate cord clamping. This has led to controversy about the timing of cord clamping at delivery (Appendix 1) but at present the evidence would suggest that clamping should be after the first minute of age in all babies who do not require resuscitation. A physiological case can be made for the cord to be clamped after the establishment of regular respirations but this has not been tested in a human trial.

Breathing at birth is stimulated by mild hypoxia and hypercarbia following cord obstruction [72, 73] as well as skin stimulation [74] and skin cooling when there is no change in core temperature [75]. If the airway is open, those first few breaths aerate the lungs [16] and continuous breathing is established. Whilst a difference in core and surface temperature may be one of the factors which stimulate the initiation of breathing, it is essential that a baby's core temperature is maintained in the normal range (Chapter 5).

Historical approaches to resuscitation

Until the late 1950's resuscitation at birth had never been subjected to systematic study. Numerous techniques such as intragastric oxygen, [3, 76, 77] the dropping of respiratory stimulant drugs on the tongue, [78-80] Eve's rocking method, [81-84] hyperbaric oxygen [85, 86] and rapid hypothermia [87, 88] were widely advocated and employed with apparent success. Though therapeutically-induced hypothermia in the post-resuscitation period has recently been shown to be useful in reducing long-term neurological damage after significant damaging hypoxia, [89-92] it is of no help during resuscitation.

All of these techniques are now discredited and several have been shown to be harmful. That more than 90% of the babies subjected to these treatments survived is a vivid testimony to the fact that most babies at birth have remarkable powers of recovery.

We now have a much better idea of what happens when mammals are subjected to acute hypoxia during birth, thanks to the work undertaken by Geoffrey Dawes in Oxford, [93] Kenneth Cross in London, [94] and a number of other neonatal physiologists, [95] and a much better idea how to respond logically and effectively. Most of what we now know about the subject was learnt between 1957 and 1967 – a decade that witnessed a complete transformation in the way newborn babies were resuscitated. That knowledge is currently being supplemented with newer techniques that enhance our understanding of the normal and abnormal transition at birth. [96]

The use of mouth-to-mouth resuscitation was first made respectable by Safar in 1958, [97] and the complementary technique of closed-chest cardiac compression was first described two years later. [98] Within a year there were reports of the latter technique being successfully used on a baby. [99] However, it took over thirty years for tracheal intubation to be widely adopted as it eventually was in the 1960's [100, 101] even though this approach had been strongly recommended by Flagg in America in 1928, [102] by Blaikley and Gibberd in England in 1935 [103], and routinely used by Virginia Apgar around 1950 [104].

Fetal response to acute hypoxia

The diagrams below (Fig 4.1 to 4.3) show data derived from animal experiments outlining the response of a mammalian fetus subjected to acute total hypoxia *in utero*. These data were obtained by opening the pregnant uterus of a mammal in such a way as to avoid uterine contraction, then preventing the fetus from being able to aerate its lungs by placing its head in a bag of saline, and finally obstructing the fetoplacental circulation. It is likely that acute intrauterine hypoxia produces similar changes in the human fetus as all mammals studied have demonstrated an identical sequence.

At the onset of acute hypoxia and hypercarbia the conscious fetus' breathing movements, driven by the respiratory centre, become deeper and more rapid. During this time the PaO_2 falls rapidly and soon the fetus loses consciousness. Within a few minutes regular breathing movements cease as the higher centres responsible for controlling them are unable to continue to function due to lack of oxygen and the fetus enters a period known as primary apnoea. Up to this point the heart rate has remained much the same but soon falls to about half its normal rate, though the blood pressure is almost unchanged.

The initial fall in heart rate is probably a vagally-induced event but this low rate is maintained because, due to lack of oxygen, the heart muscle has to function using anaerobic metabolism – a less efficient mechanism. This is possible in the newborn because the heart is packed with glycogen. Blood pressure is maintained despite a lower heart rate because vasoconstriction restricts flow to all but the most vital areas. At the same time the slower heart rate allows more time for the ventricles to refill in diastole and the stroke volume slightly increases. Overall, cardiac output drops but the fall is not as great as would be predicted from the fall in rate. By these methods circulation is maintained to the organs of the body that are most important for immediate survival but at a cost of further deterioration of the biochemical milieu with increased acidaemia due to the release of lactic acid as a by-product of anaerobic metabolism.

If the insult continues and the fetus is not delivered then, after a variable period of time, primitive spinal centres, released from suppression by the higher breathing centres, produce shuddering whole body gasps at a rate of about

12 min[-1].[93] A variable time may elapse before this unconscious gasping activity begins. Anaesthetics and drugs, especially opiates, given to the mother can increase the duration of this primary apnoeic period but the length of the following period of gasping is then reduced.[105]

During this period of gasping some cardio-pulmonary circulation is maintained but if these gasps fail to aerate the lungs they fade away as increasing acidosis and hypoxia interferes with synaptic communication between nerve cells[80] and the fetus enters terminal apnoea. Soon the rapidly deteriorating biochemical milieu due to both the metabolic and the respiratory acidosis, causes the heart muscle to cease to function effectively and, without further intervention, the baby dies. The whole process probably takes almost twenty minutes in the newborn human baby.[106]

A baby who is not breathing within a minute or two of birth could have reached one of the three points indicated by arrows in Figure 4.1. A baby born at the point indicated by the first arrow will be perfectly able to 'resuscitate' itself provided the airway is clear. After a pause this baby will take the first of a series of gasps. If the airway is open and these gasps are successful in aerating the lungs then, because the circulation is still functioning, blood newly oxygenated by the aerated lungs will be transported to the coronary arteries and the heart rate will rapidly increase.

This, in turn, will mean that oxygenated blood is transported to the brain and the respiratory centre by the improving circulation. Once the respiratory centre is functioning again, normal regular breathing will start and gasping will cease. A similar sequence of events will follow in a baby born at the second arrow, though recovery may be somewhat slower.

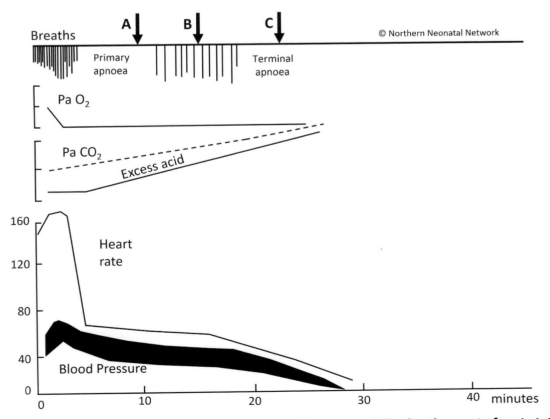

Figure 4.1 Diagrammatic representation of primary and secondary apnoea following the onset of acute total hypoxia at time 0

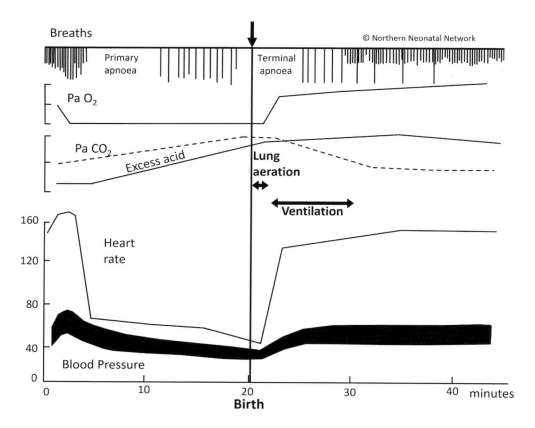

Figure 4.2 Diagrammatic representation of the physiological effect of lung aeration in a baby born in early terminal apnoea

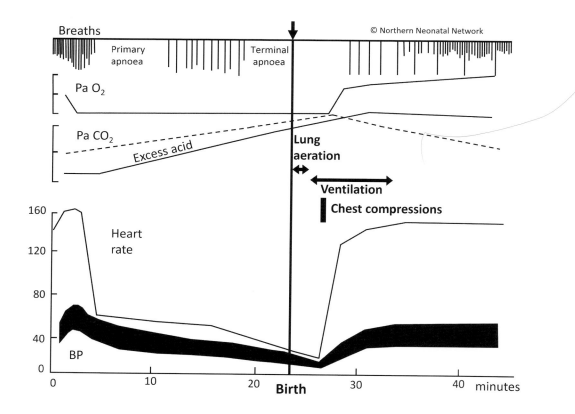

Figure 4.3 Diagrammatic representation of the physiological effect of chest compressions on a baby born in early terminal apnoea who does not respond to lung aeration and ventilation

A baby born at the point indicated by the third arrow will certainly die without intervention and may die despite it. However, effective lung aeration may be enough to produce a rapid recovery, provided the circulation is functioning sufficiently to bring some oxygenated blood back to the heart (Figure 4.2).

Unfortunately, it is not possible to tell at the time whether a baby who is not breathing at birth is in primary apnoea and about to gasp or whether it has already taken its last gasp *in utero*. It is reassuring to know, however, that almost all babies for whom help is called at birth will respond very rapidly once their lungs are aerated.

Figure 4.2 shows such a response to resuscitation from a baby in early terminal apnoea. A similar response would be expected had the baby been born in primary apnoea (arrow 1; Figure 4.1) but in that case one would expect few if any gasps following lung aeration.

In a few babies the situation may have progressed to a stage where the heart is no longer able to deliver oxygenated blood from the lungs to the coronary arteries despite adequate lung aeration with an appropriate gas. In this situation recovery may still occur in some cases if a brief period of chest compressions can successfully deliver a small quantity of oxygenated blood to the heart and provided the heart is still able to respond as is illustrated opposite (Figure 4.3). This may need to be followed by a period of intermittent positive pressure ventilation until normal breathing is established.

As previously stated, it is impossible to tell at the time whether an apnoeic baby at birth is in primary apnoea and about to gasp or whether he has already taken his last gasp *in utero* and is now in terminal apnoea. A strategy is needed which will cope equally well with either situation; such a strategy is outlined in the next chapter.

Summary learning

Most babies make the transition to extrauterine life independently and without help.

Immediate clamping of the cord may produce initial bradycardia, which then resolves.

In babies who do not require resuscitation, the cord should not be clamped for at least a minute after birth and, ideally after respirations are established.

There are three reasons why newborn babies can recover from periods of oxygen deprivation that more mature humans cannot endure:

- **In response to hypoxia the baby conserves energy by shutting down the circulation to all but the most vital organs**

- **After a latent period of so called primary apnoea, automatic, spinally-generated gasping activity appears, while at the same time.....**

- **....the heart of the term newborn baby has stores of glycogen which allows it to provide an adequate circulation in the face of considerable biochemical disturbance for a reasonably long time. This circulatory resilience is a feature of all mammals at birth.**

My key take-home messages from this chapter

The process of resuscitation at birth

Contents

- An overview of resuscitation
- Preparation for newborn resuscitation
- Additional considerations due to antenatal or intrapartum information, place of delivery, etc.
- After delivery
- Initial assessment
- Beginning resuscitation – addressing the airway and inflating (aerating) the lungs
- What to do if there is a response
- What to do if there is no response
- Teamwork, leadership and communication

Learning outcomes

To enable you to:

- **Understand how the preceding chapter on physiology relates to clinical practice**
- **Recognise the importance of preparation**
- **Consider the general approach to be adopted in resuscitation at birth**
- **Describe the logical approach to resuscitation for those few babies needing more than just gentle stimulation at birth**

Introduction

Resuscitation is likely to be rapidly successful if begun before the baby has become so hypoxic that all potential for respiratory activity has vanished. [107] Babies in primary apnoea can usually resuscitate themselves if they have a clear airway. This ability to 'self-resuscitate' is why in the past a number of unusual methods of resuscitation were promoted even though we now know them to be ineffective, and in some cases, potentially harmful.

It is not possible to determine whether an apnoeic baby at birth is in primary or secondary apnoea. A structured, staged approach to management needs to be applied that will work in either situation. This starts with thermal care and assessment then proceeds as far as necessary down the following simplified algorithm:

- Dry and cover the baby
- Assess the situation
- Airway
- Breathing
- Chest compressions
- (Drugs)

An overview of resuscitation

Dry and cover the baby

Always start by drying and covering the baby to prevent it from getting cold. A wet baby rapidly loses heat, and a small baby can quickly become dangerously hypothermic. [23] Babies subjected to cold stress in the period immediately after birth have a lower arterial oxygen tension, [24] an increased metabolic acidosis, [24] and there is evidence in animals that hypoxia, acidosis and hypothermia all tend to inhibit surfactant production. [26] Unless obviously in need of urgent attention, the baby can remain attached to the placenta during this assessment. Delayed cord clamping may confer benefit, and unless in need of immediate resuscitation, may take place on the mother's perineum or her abdomen (Appendix 1).

> **TAKE MEASURES TO MAINTAIN A BABY'S TEMPERATURE IN THE NORMAL RANGE – AVOID BOTH HYPOTHERMIA AND HYPERTHERMIA**

Assess the situation

The assessment follows a logical order; during delivery and initial handling knowledge is gained on the appearance of the baby and its tone. Whilst instituting initial thermal care observation of the chest permits an assessment of breathing. The heart rate must be actively determined, and this is best done at this stage through auscultation of the chest.

a) Airway

In order to breathe it is essential to have a clear airway otherwise air cannot be drawn into the lungs (Chapter 6). Babies in primary apnoea only require a clear airway in order to establish effective breathing (though most people would try to accelerate recovery by starting lung aeration). Provided the circulation is functioning, then oxygenated blood will be distributed to the heart and brain and in response to the oxygen the heart rate will rise.

b) Breathing

If the airway is clear and yet there is no effective breathing it is necessary to fill the lungs with air. First by inflation breaths to clear lung fluid, and then ventilation breaths (Chapter 6). In most cases the circulation is still functioning, in which case the first sign of effective oxygen delivery to the heart will be a rise in the heart rate. Breathing efforts may then improve at which point supportive ventilation might be discontinued, however some babies, particularly those who are premature, may benefit from on-going support through the use of continuous positive airway pressure (CPAP).

If the heart rate does not improve the most likely cause is failure to aerate the lungs and you should then check

whether the lungs really have been aerated by checking for chest movement. Always ensure adequate ventilation before proceeding to chest compressions. It is not usually necessary to use more than air but where the heart rate is not responding despite effective ventilation supplemental oxygen may be used.

c) Chest compressions

Where the heart rate is very slow (less than 60 min⁻¹) and there is no rise in heart rate despite adequate ventilation, as judged by visible chest movement, then the circulation may need assistance using chest compressions (Chapter 7). If correctly performed, this will bring blood from the lungs to the heart. Provided the lungs have been aerated before chest compressions are begun then the blood that returns to the heart will be oxygenated and this will usually allow the heart to respond with an increase in heart rate.

d) Drugs

In a few babies there may be no response despite good lung aeration, ventilation and effective chest compressions. This may be because of the effect of lactic acid accumulation and/or exhaustion of the limited glycogen stores in the heart muscle. In this situation reversal of the acidosis within the heart (with sodium bicarbonate), the provision of energy (with glucose) or stimulation of the myocardium (with adrenaline) may be successful, at least in theory (Chapter 7). If these drugs are used then venous access, usually via an umbilical venous catheter, will be necessary (Appendix 2).

Airway, Breathing, Chest compressions (and Drugs)

These steps must be tackled in this order (Figure 5.1). It will not be possible to aerate the lungs without a clear airway. Blood cannot be oxygenated unless air is delivered to the lungs. Chest compressions are pointless without oxygenated blood to move from the lungs to the heart.

Preparation

The need for resuscitation of the newborn infant at birth cannot always be anticipated nor predicted. Therefore, at every birth, no matter how "low risk", the birth attendants must be prepared to resuscitate the newborn infant, and know who and how to summon if further help is required.

Preparing for resuscitation requires:

- Identification of maternal, fetal and intrapartum factors that place the newborn infant at risk of requiring resuscitation.

- Communication between the person(s) caring for the mother and those responsible for receiving the newborn regarding antepartum and intrapartum factors that place the newly born infant at risk.

- Having appropriate resuscitation equipment and drugs available at all births.

- Providing a clean and warm environment for the birth.

- Skilled professional staff having appropriate qualifications and experience in newborn resuscitation – the staff that attend a birth should be trained in basic newborn resuscitation. A person trained in advanced newborn resuscitation should be available for low risk births and in attendance at all high risk births within obstetric maternity units.

- A team approach to caring for the mother and her newborn and to providing appropriate newborn resuscitation techniques, should these be needed.

If there is time:

- Introduce yourself to the parents and explain why you are there.

- Review the obstetric notes to identify any important factors (see Appendix 4 for some special considerations that may be known before delivery).

- Wash your hands, put on gloves and prepare the resuscitation area.

- Make sure any heater is on and that doors and windows are closed.

- Ensure there are enough warm towels (plastic bags for preterm babies).

- Check the gas supply and any delivery system – T-piece/mask* or bag/mask.

- Ensure air/oxygen blender* settings and pressure limits are set appropriately.

- Check that a pulse oximeter and probe are available in case they are required*.

- Check that the suction works and is set appropriately with the right type and size of catheter.

- Ensure that airway adjuncts are available – oropharyngeal airways, laryngoscope/torch.

- Check that equipment for intubation is available (if appropriate)*.

- Check venous access equipment and resuscitation drugs (if appropriate)*.

- Check the clock.

This level of equipment and expertise may not be available at home or in stand-alone midwifery unit deliveries.

Additional considerations

Sometimes the antenatal history may give information that allows you to decide whether additional help or transfer of the baby after delivery is required (see Appendix 4). In any situation always ask:

- **Do you need help?** – at all times consider whether more help is required and if so ensure it is summoned. Senior support may be needed, especially for babies 30 weeks gestation or less (Chapter 8). More staff may be needed for twins, especially if born by caesarean section; or if intra-partum monitoring suggests that the baby may have been severely compromised (e.g. a prolonged fetal bradycardia).

- **Is transport required?** – if the baby is likely to be very small or preterm then consider whether you will transfer the baby on the resuscitaire or whether you will need to arrange to have a portable incubator and air/oxygen nearby for transfer. In the home, an ambulance may need to be called.

Anticipation can often prevent difficulties. If you are attending a birth at home there can be a considerable delay between asking for help and receiving it. It is better to have help arrive and not need it than to find you really need help which has not yet been summoned.

> ## DO YOU NEED HELP?
> ## ALWAYS ASK FOR HELP IF YOU EXPECT OR ENCOUNTER ANY DIFFICULTY

After delivery

Drying and assessing the baby

- Start the clock or note the time of birth.

- Collect the baby in a warm, dry towel.

- Dry the baby promptly and effectively. Remove the wet towel and wrap in a fresh dry warm towel. (For very small or significantly preterm babies it is better to place the wet baby in a polythene bag or wrap – and place under a radiant heater). Cover the head with a hat or towel.

- During this period it is possible to assess the baby and decide whether any intervention is going to be needed. For apparently well babies there is no need to rush to clamp the cord. Unless the baby is clearly in need of immediate resuscitation, wait for at least one minute from the complete delivery of the baby before clamping the cord. Keep the baby warm during this time.

If the baby is thought to need assistance then this becomes the priority. In order to provide assistance the baby may need to be moved; which in turn may involve disconnecting the baby from the placenta. If the baby is limp or very pale, has a very slow heart rate (less than 60 min^{-1}) or is making no effort to breathe then transfer the baby to the resuscitation area.

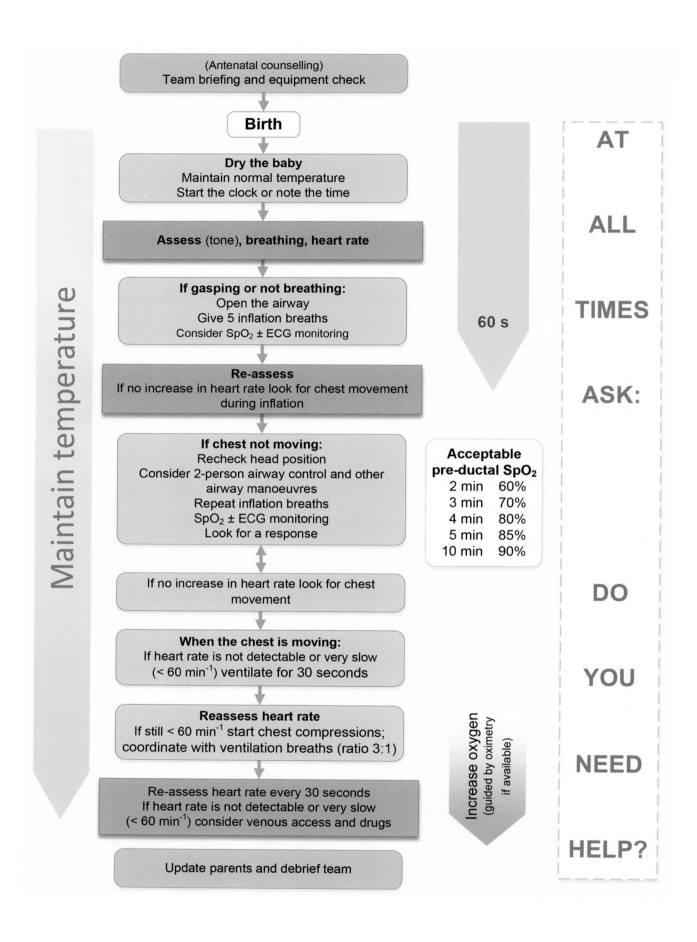

Figure 5.1 Newborn Life Support Algorithm

Stimulation

The process of delivery will often stimulate the baby, as will the subsequent handling and drying. This is usually sufficient.

Initial assessment

The initial assessment is a clinical one and usually undertaken without the use of monitors. You need to assess the baby's:

Colour
Tone
Breathing
Heart Rate

Colour: colour does not appear in the algorithm (figure 5.1) because it is not as good a means of assessing oxygenation, nor is it a reliable means of assessing how this is improving during resuscitation, as was often previously thought. [108] However, it is mentioned here because it is still thought to be useful for assessing the initial condition of the baby at birth. Babies in difficulties because of acidosis or serious blood loss will appear very pale at birth whereas the more normal colour is blue. Very pale babies who remain pale after resuscitation may be hypovolaemic as well as acidotic.

Tone: babies born well-flexed and with good tone are usually fine. A baby who is very floppy is unconscious and in significant difficulties. The tone of a baby is often clear from its posture but can also be rapidly assessed by handling the baby.

Breathing: breathing usually starts spontaneously within a minute of birth and whilst apnoea on assessment may warrant action it is important to realise that some perfectly healthy babies can take up to three minutes to start breathing after birth. [46] The baby may show normal regular breaths, irregular breaths, gasping (sometimes interspersed amongst more normal breaths), or breathing may be absent (apnoea).

Gasping breaths are usually accompanied by recession but recession is also occasionally seen with regular breathing, suggesting increased work of breathing. This may be due to partial obstruction of the airway or stiff lungs in premature babies.

Heart rate: in healthy term babies the heart rate is usually greater than 100 min⁻¹ by 2 min of age but can be still below that rate at 3 min in about 10%.[49] In well preterm babies this proportion is slightly greater. Similarly, in term infants in whom cord clamping is delayed, the additional blood volume leads to a less dramatic change in heart rate and 10% of babies still have a heart rate less than 100 min⁻¹ after 5 min (these infants are otherwise healthy). [109]

Assessing the heart rate can be done in several ways:

- **Using a stethoscope:** when first assessing the heart rate use a stethoscope. It is usually clear whether the

heart rate is very slow (less than 60 min⁻¹), slow (60–100 min⁻¹) or fast (more than 100 min⁻¹). It is not necessary to count it with complete accuracy

The cardiac impulse may often be felt at the umbilicus or the apex. However it cannot always be felt, and the rate judged by cord pulsation, if slow, may not reflect the true heart rate [47]

- **ECG monitoring:** this has recently been demonstrated to rapidly and accurately determine the heart rate at birth. [110] A reliable ECG signal can be obtained more quickly than a pulse oximetry signal, however it only registers the electrical heart beat (i.e. there is an electrical signal), not whether there is any effective output [111]

- **Pulse oximetry:** attempting to judge oxygenation by assessing skin colour is unreliable [108] but it is still worth noting the baby's colour at birth as well as whether, when and how it changes

Using a pulse oximeter will allow accurate assessment of heart rate and oxygen saturation within about two minutes of application (Appendix 3). Saturation levels in healthy babies in the first few minutes of life may be considerably lower than at other times. [112] In babies at birth the arterial oxygen saturation may be different depending on whether it is measured in areas supplied by blood leaving the aorta before or after the entry of the arterial duct (i.e. whether they are pre-ductal or post-ductal measurements). Measurements taken in the right arm are pre-ductal whereas measurements from other limbs will be post-ductal. The values quoted in the tables in this manual are all right arm (pre-ductal) values.

Values in the table below are taken from babies of **all** gestations in a study of over 450 healthy babies who received no resuscitation and no additional oxygen in the minutes immediately after birth. The data came from 308 term babies, 121 babies between 32 and 36 weeks gestation and 39 babies under 32 weeks gestation. [112]

The saturation levels listed in Table 5.1 are deemed 'acceptable' in the sense that babies exhibiting these levels probably do not need any supplemental oxygen. However, babies whose saturation levels are significantly lower *might* warrant careful supplementation. Babies with oxygen saturations of 95% or more do not need added oxygen.

Time from birth	Acceptable (25th centile) right arm saturation (%)
2 min	60
3 min	70
4 min	80
5 min	85
10 min	90

Table 5.1 Acceptable right arm oxygen saturations after birth

A pulse oximeter can be very helpful in giving an accurate readout of heart rate and also has the advantage of giving information on oxygen saturation. If you don't have a pulse oximeter or an ECG, a stethoscope is the most reliable means of monitoring heart rate.

If a baby has reasonable tone, and otherwise appears well despite a slow heart rate, then it is reasonable to wait a minute or so, whilst ensuring that the baby's head is appropriately positioned (see below).

If the baby has a good heart rate and is making good respiratory effort then no further help is required. Once wrapped, this baby should be given to the mother.

Airway opening manoeuvres

If a baby is not breathing adequately, or is gasping, then the first step is to open the airway. The airway may be obstructed if the neck is either too flexed or too extended or - in a floppy baby on its back - if the tongue falls back into the airway due to loss of pharyngeal tone (Chapter 6). These mechanisms are more likely to be the cause of an airway problem than any mechanical obstruction from blood, thick mucus, or lumps of vernix or meconium.

After opening the airway and stimulation some babies start to make satisfactory breathing efforts in which case continue to support the airway, and observe. Reassess the heart rate to ensure this is satisfactory. No other action may be required.

Meconium: most babies born through meconium stained liquor have not inhaled any particulate material into the lower respiratory tract. If they have not done so as a result of anoxic gasping before birth they will only very rarely do so at birth. [113] Suction of the baby's airways on the perineum or routine suction after delivery are not recommended but if a baby is born floppy, unresponsive and covered in thick meconium the upper airway may **quickly** be inspected under direct vision and the oropharynx cleared of material which might obstruct. However, in a bradycardic baby the emphasis **must** be to inflate the lungs within the first minute after birth and this should not be delayed. There is no evidence to support routine tracheal suctioning in this situation unless there is evidence that the trachea is blocked. [114]

> ### SCREAMING BABIES HAVE AN OPEN AIRWAY
>
> ### FLOPPY BABIES – HAVE A QUICK LOOK IN THE OROPHARYNX;
>
> ### BUT DO NOT DELAY LUNG INFLATION

Inflation breaths

In order to clear lung fluid in an unresponsive baby, positive pressure inflations with a long inspiration time are required (Chapter 6). For a term baby, start at pressures of about 30 cm water [115] with inflation times sustained for 2-3 s. [116] Five such 'inflation breaths' should be sufficient to aerate the lung. Significantly preterm babies (30 weeks and below) may well respond to a lower initial inflation pressure of 20–25 cm water (Chapter 8). [117-119] In all babies it is reasonable to start resuscitation with air (21% oxygen) but in significantly preterm babies (30 weeks and below) a starting range of 21-30% oxygen may be used.

Having given five inflation breaths – reassess to see if the baby has responded.

Reassess – has the heart rate improved?

Heart rate *is* increasing

If inflation breaths have aerated the lungs you would expect the heart rate to increase within 5–10 s. This is one of the first signs that the baby is responding. If the heart rate is increasing rapidly then you can assume that you have successfully aerated the lungs. You then proceed as follows:

- **Ventilation support:** following inflation breaths the baby may start breathing spontaneously. If this does not occur, gently ventilate the lungs at about 30 breaths min[-1] until the baby starts to breathe. If your ventilation is adequate the heart rate will remain above 100 beats min[-1]. If it falls below this it suggests that your ventilation is inadequate. Recheck the airway position and ventilation technique. Pressures of ~20 cm water and inspiratory times of less than 1 s are usually adequate for ventilation once the lungs have been inflated

- **Reassess - is there spontaneous breathing?** With continued support, breathing efforts will usually return. The manner in which these return is important. If the first efforts are gasping in nature, this would suggest that the baby may have been in terminal apnoea. It is important to record the sequence and timing of events. If the heart rate is satisfactory but no spontaneous breathing returns then you might consider other factors such as sedation, neurological issues or intrathoracic pathology. Remember, it is possible to render a healthy baby apnoeic by lowering the $PaCO_2$ with hyperventilation

Heart rate *is not* increasing

If the heart rate **is not** responding the **most likely reason** is that you have failed to aerate the lungs. Go back and check airway-opening manoeuvres and repeat the inflation breaths.

This is the time at which to consider using two-person airway support and other airway manoeuvres (Chapter 6).

- **Reassess – is there chest movement?** In the absence of a heart rate response, seeing the chest move as you give inflation breaths is the only way to judge successful aeration of the lungs. Listening for breath sounds with a stethoscope can be misleading because of transmitted upper airway sounds. Chest movement may only start to occur after the first few (two or three) effective inflation breaths. Check for chest movement as you give a further set of inflation breaths. Once you have confirmed chest movement ventilate for 30 s and then reassess.

- **Reassess – is the heart rate satisfactory?** If the heart rate remains slow or absent, despite adequate ventilation as shown by chest movement, then you need to give chest compressions (Chapter 7). Chest compressions should help to move oxygenated blood from the lungs to the heart and coronary arteries. The blood you move can only be oxygenated if the lungs have air in them.

- **Reassess – has the heart rate improved?** It is usually only necessary to continue chest compressions for about 20–30 s before the heart responds with an increase in heart rate [13].

- **Consider drugs:** if the baby has subjected to severe hypoxic stress then these simple measures may not be enough to produce an increase in heart rate. In this situation it may be necessary to use drugs to alter the intracardiac milieu or to stimulate the heart. The venous access necessary to give these drugs is most easily achieved using an umbilical venous catheter (Chapter 7 and Appendix 2).

- **Reassess – has the heart rate improved?** If the heart rate is still not improving consider other factors such as hypovolaemia, tension pneumothorax, diaphragmatic hernia or, rarely, complete heart block.

- **Reassess – should resuscitation attempts continue?** If there was no detectable heart rate at birth and still none by ten minutes of age, survival is unlikely and long-term serious neurological disability amongst the rare survivors is very likely. It is entirely appropriate to consider

stopping at this point (Chapter 11). [17, 18] If the heart rate remains slow at 10 min and is not improving the outlook is still very poor but the situation is more complex and senior advice should be urgently sought.

Teamwork, leadership and communication

In the majority of cases simple resuscitation measures result in a speedy recovery and in most cases additional help is not required. In a minority of cases additional help is required and to be effective any intervention needs the right people to be working together in the right place at the right time, and with the right equipment. How this is achieved is discussed in Chapter 12.

In an emergency, structured communication helps.
Communication problems are a factor in up to 80% of adverse incidents or near miss reports in hospitals. This failure of communication is also evident when a newborn emergency occurs and a doctor, nurse or midwife summons senior help. The caller often fails to communicate the seriousness of the situation or conveys the information in a way that fails to ensure that the recipient appreciates the urgency of the situation. A well-structured process that is simple, reliable and dependable will enable the caller to convey the important facts, the degree of urgency and allow the recipient to plan ahead.

Use of the acronym SBAR (Situation-Background-Assessment-Recommendation) is now widely accepted across the health service can be helpful in planning effective, timely communication between individuals from different clinical backgrounds and hierarchies.

SBAR	Content	Example A	Example B
Situation	Introduce yourself and check you are speaking to the correct person Identify the patient you are calling about (who and where) State what you need	I am the senior midwife on the labour ward I am calling about Ms Smith There is cord prolapse and we are proceeding to immediate section	I am the senior midwife on the labour ward I am calling about baby Smith in room five The baby is grunting at one hour of age
Background	Important features of pregnancy and delivery Term or preterm Condition at birth and response to any resuscitation	Pregnancy has been normal This is a term labour that was normal until the membranes ruptured five minutes ago The umbilical cord has prolapsed	Pregnancy has been normal Delivery was by elective section for breech at 38 weeks The baby was in good condition at birth and did not need resuscitation, but has been grunting since 10 minutes of age
Assessment	**Undelivered mother** Progression of labour, CTG findings **Baby** Colour, Tone, Breathing, Heart rate	The cord is in the vagina It is still pulsating	Baby is pink in air, HR is >100, tone is normal, RR is 60 per minute with grunting
Recommendation	State explicitly what you want the person you are calling to do What by when?	Please attend theatre one immediately Please alert your seniors	I am not too concerned, but I would like you to review the baby within 30 minutes

Summary learning

- **The approach to newborn resuscitation follows a standard algorithm:**
  - **Dry and cover the baby**
  - **Assess the situation**
  - **Airway**
  - **Breathing – inflation breaths**
  - **Chest compressions**
  - **(Drugs).**
- **Preparation is an essential component of successful resuscitation.**
- **Most babies respond quickly to simple basic life support.**
- **More complicated and prolonged resuscitation requires teamwork, leadership and effective communication.**

My key take-home messages from this chapter

Airway management and ventilation

Contents

- **Anatomical considerations**
- **Opening the airway**
- **Head position**
- **Aerating the lungs**
- **Choosing and applying a mask**
- **Holding the facemask**
- **What to do if there is no response**
- **Difficult airways and situations (including tracheal obstruction and meconium)**
- **Oxygen and monitoring**
- **Airway adjuncts**

Learning outcomes

To enable you to:

- **Consider why babies might not be able to breathe**
- **Understand the theory of airway management and positive pressure ventilation using a facemask**
- **Describe the equipment available to manage an airway, its advantages and limitations**
- **Adopt a structured approach to managing the airway in a newborn baby and how to provide respiratory support to that baby when it is not breathing or the breathing is inadequate**
- **Discuss strategies for coping with more difficult and complex airway problems**

Introduction

Management of the airway and support of breathing are two of the most important skills required in helping babies at birth. This chapter discusses the two key elements:

- how to open an airway, and, once open,

- how to aerate the lungs and support breathing (if this is required) once the airway is open.

The majority of babies do not need help with breathing at birth; a small number, however, do. The most commonly encountered scenario is the hypoxic baby who has become unconscious and as a result has lost its respiratory drive, and has floppy obstructed airways. Other scenarios (Table 6.1) are less common, although the approach to each is similar.

NLS

1. Loss of respiratory drive

- Acquired depression of the neurological centres responsible for initiating breathing in the unconscious baby
  - perinatal stress & hypoxia
  - drugs e.g. maternal sedation/analgesia
  - infection
- Congenital brain abnormality

2. Mechanical obstruction of the airway

- Loss of muscular tone affecting patency of the airway
  - unconscious baby
  - congenital conditions affecting muscles
- Foreign body
  - meconium, vernix, blood, mucus plug
- Anatomical abnormality of the airway (e.g. Pierre-Robin Sequence)

3. Inability to breathe

- Neurological and muscular conditions affecting the ability to breathe

Table 6.1: Reasons for difficulties with breathing at birth.

Anatomical Considerations

The airway of a newborn baby is different to the adult airway in ways which make it more vulnerable to mechanical obstruction. The tongue is proportionally larger, taking up more space in the mouth. The larynx is more anterior and the pharynx tapered towards the cords like a funnel. In the unconscious baby with reduced tone, and who is placed on their back, the pharynx has a tendency to collapse and both the jaw and tongue to fall back obstructing the airway.

Matters are further compounded by the shape of the newborn head. The occiput is relatively large – especially after a normal delivery where cranial moulding exaggerates the tendency. The large occiput causes the neck to flex when the baby is placed supine on a flat surface – further compressing airway structures and obstructing the airway.

Opening the airway

The obstruction caused by the tendency of the pharynx to collapse and the tongue to fall back obstructing the airway in the unconscious or obtunded baby lying on its back can be overcome by lifting the jaw (and thus the base of the tongue) forward. Two manoeuvres can be used to ensure an open airway in an unconscious baby:

1. Hold the head in the neutral position with chin and jaw support.
2. Move the jaw forward using a two-handed jaw thrust.

> **MASK INFLATION WILL NOT WORK UNLESS THE AIRWAY IS OPEN**

Head position

To overcome the tendency of the neck to flex due to the prominence of the occiput when the floppy newborn baby is placed on its back (supine) you should place the baby's head in the neutral position with the neck neither extended nor flexed (Figure 6.1). If the baby is on a flat surface then the neutral position can be easily achieved by placing a small (~2 cm thick) pad under the baby's shoulders.

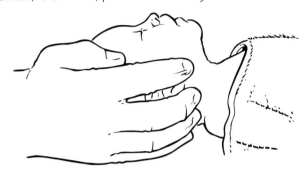

Figure 6.1 Hold the head in the neutral position.

Perhaps the most common reason for failure to open the airway is incorrect positioning of the neck – usually over extension.

Chin support and jaw thrust

In a baby with poor tone who is breathing it will be necessary to support the chin using a finger on the bony part of the chin near the tip (Figure 6.2). Avoid pressing on the soft tissue under the chin as this may push the tongue base backwards and worsen the situation. If the baby is very floppy it may be necessary to use one or two fingers under each side of the lower jaw at its angle to push the jaw forwards (Figure 6.3). This requires two hands but it is the most effective method of jaw thrust. If a mask is applied to the face the jaw must always be supported by either chin support or jaw thrust.

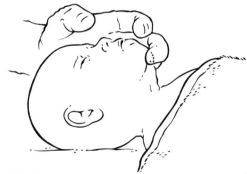

Figure 6.2 Chin support

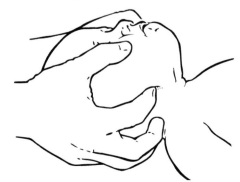

Figure 6.3 Jaw thrust

NLS

NEWBORN LIFE SUPPORT

In the conscious, or semi-conscious, baby who is trying to breathe, the manoeuvres described above may be sufficient to enable the baby to cope. If the heart rate is adequate, no further intervention may be necessary. If the baby is **not** breathing, then the situation will not improve without additional intervention. The baby needs help with lung inflation and breathing.

Aerating the lungs

Until the baby takes its first breath the lungs are filled with fluid. In fetal life the lung secretes large quantities of lung fluid which pass out into the amniotic cavity. [67] In all mammals studied the volume of fluid in the lungs at birth is about 30 mL kg^{-1} – this equates to ~100 mL in the average term baby. At the onset of normal labour various hormonal changes result in cells within the fetal lung switching from secreting to absorbing fluid. [120] A small amount of fluid, perhaps 35 mL or so in a term baby, is expelled via the oropharynx during the passage through the birth canal but once breathing starts about 70 mL [15, 120] is rapidly reabsorbed into the blood stream and the lymphatics within a few minutes. [16] This process is augmented by the inflation of the lungs themselves. [121] Babies who are born by caesarean section prior to the onset of labour will not have had the opportunity to 'prepare' their lungs in this way and this may go some way to explaining why such babies have a higher incidence of respiratory problems. [122]

Healthy, vigorous babies can achieve lung aeration with their first breath using negative pressures of around minus 30 cm water, but frequently less than minus 20 cm water. [123] Well babies can achieve a resting lung volume of 15–30 mL with the first breath. Once a breath has been taken intrathoracic pressure is then often raised, by crying, to levels of 30–90 cm water. This probably helps to move lung fluid into the pulmonary interstitial tissues during the first few breaths. [124]

Babies needing resuscitation at birth need help in achieving a resting lung volume. If positive pressure ventilation is used then a relatively long inspiration time of 2–3 s [116] is required to aerate the lung of a newborn baby. When ventilating using positive pressure ventilation gas will not enter the lung until it reaches a pressure above the so-called 'opening pressure' of the lung. Theoretical calculations from measurements in isolated lungs as well as data from newborn babies would suggest that the opening pressure in babies needing resuscitation is 15-30 cm water (1.5-2.9 kPa) with a mean of about 20. [125]

In term babies needing resuscitation we therefore recommend using an inflation pressure of 30 cm water. Some suggest using a higher pressure because a higher flow rate will result. However, lung aeration depends on the volume of gas delivered which is a function of both flow and time. A lower pressure (if higher than the opening pressure) will be just as effective as a higher pressure, if applied for a longer time. Though a pressure of 40 cm water sustained for half a second can be effective [126], an inflation pressure of 30 cm water applied for 2–3 s (and repeated five times) will adequately aerate the lungs of most babies at birth and this is the recommended approach. [106, 126, 127]

Facemask aeration and ventilation using a self-inflating bag as a source of pressurised gas is a skill that should be acquired by all involved in the care of the newborn. It can be difficult to do well, however, and requires practice. [128] Using a facemask with a T-piece, a continuous supply of gas and a pressure-limiting device is generally felt to be easier, but requires a source of pressurised gas. This method was first described in 1913 and has been 'rediscovered' on many occasions since. [129-132]

The essential pre-requisites for **both** techniques are:

- an open airway

- a good seal between the mask and the baby's face.

Choosing and applying a mask

It is easiest to obtain a seal with a silicone mask with a broad, soft deformable sealing surface or flange but anatomical masks with a cushion can work as well (Figure 6.4a). [133-136]

The soft deformable flange of a silicone mask is designed to mould around the baby's face to create an airtight seal during application of positive pressure. When such masks are applied to the face, force should be applied down through the mask with fingers holding the thickened upper section and avoiding the rim – which if squeezed may deform to break the seal against the face. Beware of applying excessive force – which may be uncomfortable for the baby and also deform the mask and create a less effective seal.

Other masks have a rigid upper section and a soft inflatable cushion. It is important to ensure the cushion is inflated, but not excessively so. Once again, the mask is held by the rigid upper section and it is the force applied through the mask which pushes the cushion against the face to make a seal.

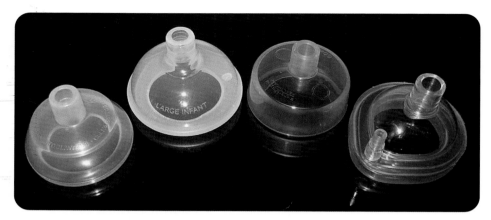

Figure 6.4a Commonly used facemasks for term babies from different manufacturers. From left to right; silicone round facemask (reusable), silicone round domed facemask (single-use), round silicone facemask (single-use), anatomical facemask with rigid upper section and inflatable rim (single-use).

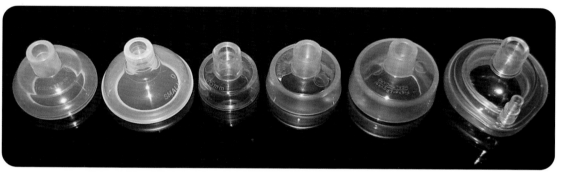

Figure 6.4b Common preterm mask designs showing variation in sizes.

The mask should cover the nose and mouth but should not extend over the edge of the chin and nor should it encroach on the orbits. Failure to achieve an airtight seal between the mask and the face is a common reason for failure of mask ventilation. Not surprising then that small babies need small masks (Figure 6.4b).

After correctly sizing the mask there are three key ways (3 P's) to reduce mask leak and achieve a virtually air-tight seal:

1. **POSITION:** Rolling the mask onto the face ("align, roll, check") for a correct mask *position* (Figure 6.5a–b).

2. **PRESSURE:** Balancing the *pressure* exerted on the mask by the finger and thumb (Figure 6.6).

3. **PULL:** Lifting or *pulling* the jaw upwards into the mask (Figure 6.7).

These three steps used correctly can ensure that an effective mask seal is created; they can be applied to any mask design, term and preterm resuscitation and single resuscitator or two-person techniques.

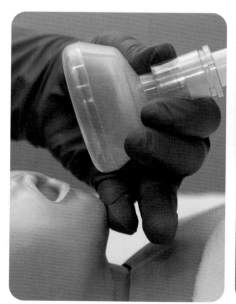 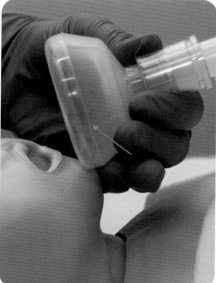 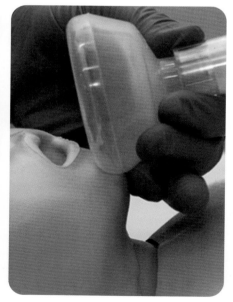

(a) Finger providing chin support   (b) Identify the demarcating line   (c) Align line with chin tip

Fig 6.5a *Align* the mask on the chin tip

NLS

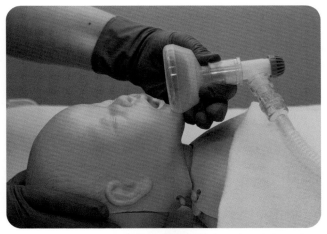

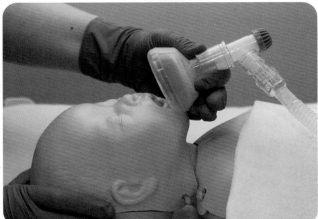

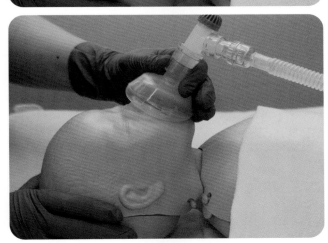

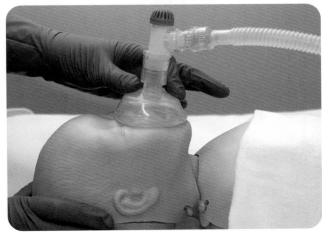

Figure 6.5b Carefully *roll* the mask upwards

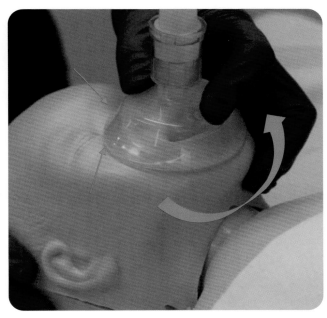

Figure 6.6 Carefully *check* the mask position and balance pressure exerted on the mask by the finger and thumb

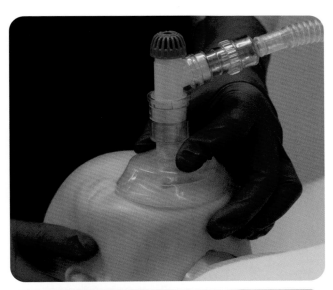

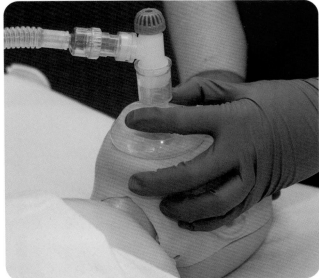

Figure 6.7 Apply jaw lift (Pulling the jaw up into the mask)

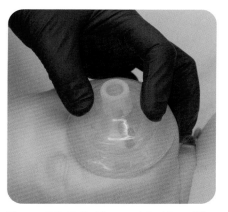 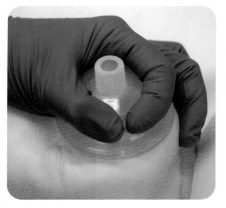 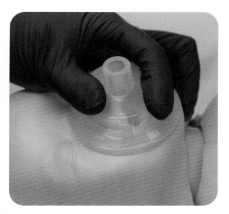

Figure 6.8 Suitable mask hold positions. From left to right; the two point top hold, the encircling hold and the C-grip hold.

Having done this:

- re-check the 3 P's: **Position**, **Pressure**, **Pulling** the jaw up
- re-check the airway position: is the head still in the neutral position?
- then give inflation breaths.

Holding the facemask

There are a number of ways to hold the facemask (Figure 6.8), the key attributes of all these methods is that they ensure even pressure on the top of the mask without deforming the cuff of the silicone type masks. [137]

If the operator's hands are of sufficient size, then placing the thenar eminence (heel of the hand) on the forehead of the baby helps achieve stability.

Give inflation breaths

To aerate the lungs give five inflation breaths, sustaining the inflation pressure at about 30 cm water for 2–3 s with each breath. Too low a pressure is ineffective and too high a pressure can be dangerous. If there is a blender in the circuit it should usually be set to **AIR** in the first instance (or air-30% oxygen for babies of 30 weeks gestation or less).

The first two or three breaths will merely replace fluid with air without changing the volume of the chest. Therefore you would not expect the chest to move until the fourth or fifth breath. After the first five inflations the lungs will be aerated and further ventilation can be managed with lower pressures (see below).

Lung aeration is more easily achieved with a constant-flow pressure-limited device, such as a T-piece system, than a volume limited device such as a self-inflating bag. Sustained pressure is necessary to expand the lungs of the unconscious baby at birth, and this is less easily achieved with self-inflating bag-mask systems. [128, 138, 139] However, whilst self-inflating bags and T-Piece systems have been found equally effective clinically, [140, 141] self-inflating bags are not as effective at delivering positive end expiratory pressure (PEEP), consistent peak pressures or inspiratory times. [142, 143]

Intubation (Appendix 2) can provide a secure airway and

once fixed in place, frees the hands to concentrate on circulatory resuscitation if that is needed. However, the tracheal tube must be the correct diameter, the correct length, and securely fixed in the correct orifice. If any of these are not done properly then mask ventilation is likely to be more effective.

> **AERATE THE LUNGS WITH FIVE 'INFLATION BREATHS' USING 30 CM WATER PRESSURE EACH BREATH APPLIED FOR 2-3 S**

Check for a response

If you have successfully aerated the lungs and if the heart can respond then you will detect an increase in the baby's heart rate within 30 s. Therefore, if an increase in the heart rate is detected and maintained you can assume lung aeration has been successful.

> **THE FIRST RESPONSE TO SUCCESSFUL LUNG INFLATION AND AERATION IS AN INCREASE IN HEART RATE**

If the heart rate **does not** increase, this usually means that you have not successfully aerated the lungs. In some cases, however, it may mean that you have aerated the lungs but the heart cannot respond. If the heart rate does not respond to inflation breaths the only way to check that the lungs have been aerated successfully is to see the chest move in response to your inflation breaths.

If the heart rate increases

If the heart rate has increased satisfactorily, then interventions have been successful, and no further inflation breaths are required. If the baby is not breathing, continued respiratory support with **ventilation** breaths are needed.

No increase in heart rate? – look for chest movement

If you **have** seen chest movement during your inflation breaths and the heart rate has not increased then deliver *ventilation* breaths at a rate of 30 min⁻¹ and then reassess.

If you **have not** seen chest movement, repeat the *inflation* breaths paying close attention to the chest movement. If you do not see chest movement after another five inflation breaths the most likely reason is that the airway is obstructed either because the head is not in the neutral position or because the jaw has not been drawn forwards. Two-person airway control or an oropharyngeal (Guedel) airway can be very helpful at this point. Only very occasionally is the airway blocked by mucus, vernix, blood or meconium.

When trying to inflate or ventilate the lungs always be mindful of the position of the baby's head and jaw. Any baby hypoxic enough to require urgent resuscitation is likely to be unconscious and as limp as a patient under general anaesthesia, so the airway needs to be guarded and maintained. Use the airway opening manoeuvres described previously and recheck the position.

If you do not have a second person to help then check the head is in the neutral position in case it has moved; ensure that adequate jaw thrust has been provided and repeat the five inflation breaths.

> **IF THERE IS NO VISIBLE CHEST MOVEMENT THEN THERE MAY HAVE BEEN NO LUNG INFLATION.**
>
> **REPOSITION AND REPEAT 5 INFLATION BREATHS.**
>
> **ALWAYS CHECK FOR A RESPONSE AFTER EVERY MANOEUVRE**

If you do not see chest movement after another five inflation breaths the most likely reason is that the airway is obstructed either because the head is still not in the neutral position or because the jaw has not been drawn forwards. At this stage other manoeuvres need to be considered.

Use two people (two-person airway support)

It is much easier to give mask inflation with two people. [144] One person stands (or kneels) at the baby's head holding the head in the neutral position applies jaw thrust and concentrates on making a good seal with the mask. The second person occludes the T-piece or squeezes the bag. The two techniques for holding the facemask are shown in Figure 6.9.

Use an oropharyngeal airway

An oropharyngeal airway (Guedel) should always be available and these are especially useful if there is some oro-facial abnormality affecting the airway. This can happen with a cleft palate – especially if there is micrognathia – or where the nasal passages are blocked or have not formed as in choanal atresia. Airways can also be helpful when you are having difficulty providing both jaw thrust and mask inflation on your own and help is not immediately available. Under these circumstances an airway of the appropriate size will perform the same task as jaw thrust – that is support the tongue forwards out of the oropharynx.

Choosing an oropharyngeal airway

When using an oropharyngeal airway it is important to choose the correct size. When held along the line of the lower jaw with the flange in the middle of the lips (immediately below the tip of the nose), the end of the airway should reach the angle of the jaw (Figure 6.10).

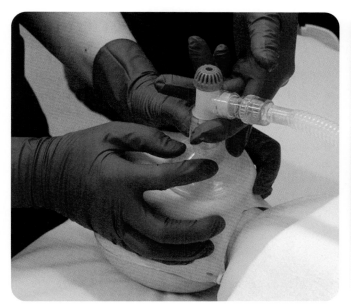

Four-point top-hold with jaw support

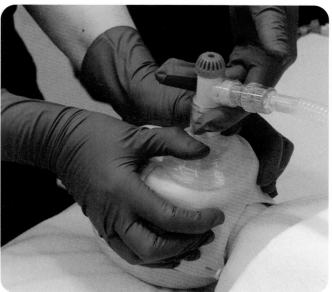

Two-thumb hold with jaw support

Figure 6.9 Face mask ventilation using two people

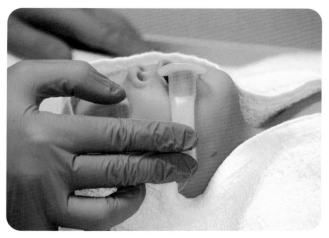

Figure 6.10 Choosing the appropriate size of oropharyngeal airway

In babies and young children the airway is inserted in the same attitude that it will finally lie. Ideally, insertion should be done under direct vision with the aid of a laryngoscope or tongue depressor to hold the tongue (Figure 6.11). Make sure that the airway slips over the tongue and does not push the tongue backwards into the back of the mouth.

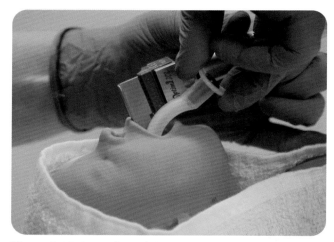

Figure 6.11 Insertion of the oropharyngeal airway using a laryngoscope

Sizing the oropharyngeal airway as above is only approximate and an assessment will also need to be made as the airway is inserted. Babies can vary in size from less than 500 to over 5000 g whereas there are only three sizes of oropharyngeal airway, 4, 5 and 6 cm. If the airway is too short the distal end will impact on the base of the tongue and may be occluded. If the airway is too long it may extend into the oropharynx below the tracheal opening and might obstruct the airway itself. The ideal length will reach just beyond the base of the tongue and will not protrude far out of the mouth in the unconscious baby.

Once inserted, reapply the face mask as previously described, re-establish the neutral position and give

another five inflation breaths. Look for chest movement and check for an increase in heart rate.

If an airway is being considered, then it is both logical and pragmatic to have a look in the oropharynx at the same time as the laryngoscope is being used to control the tongue to exclude physical obstruction by particulate matter.

Inspection under direct vision & suction

The airway is usually clear but if in doubt consider gentle direct examination of the mouth and oropharynx using a laryngoscope. The airway can be blocked by particulate matter such as meconium, vernix, blood or mucus. Any of these may be inhaled by the gasping baby *in utero* or during delivery resulting in airway compromise.

Do not blindly insert a suction catheter into the mouth. Stimulation in the region of the posterior pharynx and larynx should be kept to a minimum because it easily induces adduction of the vocal cords and profound vagal bradycardia (though it will have little effect in a baby in terminal apnoea). Very rarely the trachea may be obstructed by particulate matter aspirated before delivery or even after delivery. This can only be cleared by tracheal intubation and suction.

Equipment for positive pressure ventilation

> **NEVER CONNECT A BABY DIRECTLY TO A WALL OR CYLINDER-MOUNTED FLOWMETER WITHOUT A SUITABLE BLOW-OFF VALVE IN THE CIRCUIT**

T-piece

A soft close-fitting facemask, a supply of piped air, and a suitable pressure release valve (preferably adjustable) are all that are needed (Figure 6.12). A small pressure dial in the circuit is a useful 'optional extra', however, many would suggest that its inclusion is essential. This may indicate that a good seal has been achieved if the needle rises to the set pressure but is not completely reliable in this regard. Most T-piece circuits are now able to provide PEEP.

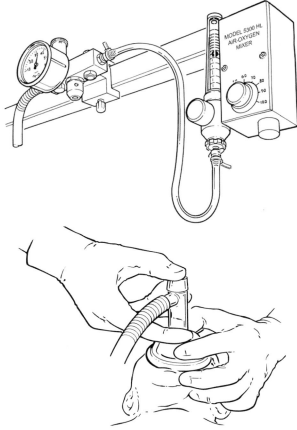

Figure 6.12 A T-piece system showing air-oxygen blender (top right), manometer and blow-off valve (top left) and use with facemask

Self-inflating 'bag-mask' system

These can be used in much the same way where there is no piped gas, but are generally more difficult to use. Self-inflating bags are discussed in more detail in Appendix 3.

Difficult airways and situations

When attempting lung inflation if the heart rate remains slow, and the chest does not move then the **AIRWAY** is the problem. When the more common causes (described above) have been ruled out consider tracheal obstruction even in the absence of meconium.

Tracheal obstruction

It is rare for tracheal obstruction to occur at delivery. However, it is very important to develop a logical approach to resuscitation and to bear this rare, but important, complication in mind. Reports of a court case from 2008 concerning this complication are very instructive. [145-147]

A baby gasping *in utero* or during delivery can inhale debris deep into the trachea. This can then block the trachea, frustrating attempts at lung inflation. It is important to be aware that meconium is not the only substance that can do this. A blood clot, a lump of thick vernix or viscid mucus or any other particulate matter, if large enough, can also cause obstruction in the trachea.

Aspirating the trachea

Material thick enough to cause airway obstruction cannot be sucked up any catheter small enough to be passed down inside a tracheal tube. The whole tracheal tube should be used as a suction device (Figure 6.13). Otherwise use the widest bore suction catheter available – preferably a 12 or 14 French gauge suction catheter passed directly into the trachea.

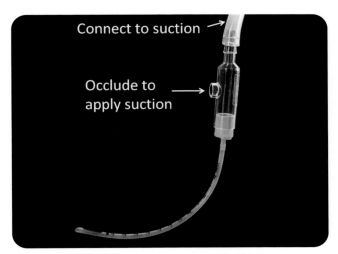

Figure 6.13 With a suitable adaptor (in this case a meconium aspirator) a tracheal tube can be used as a suction catheter

Meconium

Lightly meconium stained liquor is common and does not usually give rise to much difficulty during transition. The much less common finding of very thick or particulate meconium stained liquor at birth is an indicator of perinatal distress. The normal gentle 'breathing' efforts of a baby *in utero* are not sufficient to inhale particulate meconium in significant quantities. It is therefore reasonable to assume that if a baby has inhaled significant quantities of particulate meconium *in utero* then that baby has been gasping. In other words, that baby has been insulted to such an extent that it has passed through primary apnoea and into the gasping phase before delivery. If that is the case then the major determinants of the outcome for that baby are the circumstances and severity of the hypoxic insult that caused the baby to gasp rather than the meconium inhaled as a result of the gasping. This may be why several observational studies [113, 148-154] and two recent small randomised trials [114, 155] of intubation and suction of the airways of ***non-breathing*** babies born through meconium-stained liquor have shown no benefit to this practice. Prolonged partial hypoxia can cause hyper-reactivity of the pulmonary vasculature and, in severe cases, excessive muscularisation within pulmonary vessels, resulting in persistent fetal circulation, pulmonary vascular necrosis and haemorrhage. [156]

Most babies born from meconium-stained liquor have not inhaled any particulate material into the lower respiratory tract. If they have not done so as a result a period of

NLS

anoxic gasping before birth they will only very rarely do so at birth. [113] Large, multi-centre randomised studies have shown that the previously advocated practice of aspirating the airways of the emerging baby before delivery followed by intubation and suction of the trachea after delivery – the so-called 'combined obstetric and paediatric approach' – is not effective and does not prevent the development of meconium aspiration syndrome. [113, 148-154, 157, 158] Moreover there was increasing evidence suggesting that attempting to inspect the oropharynx or even intubate vigorous term babies was harmful. However, it is worth remembering that meconium is only one of several substances (also blood, thick mucous, vernix) that may on rare occasions cause tracheal obstruction.

The approach to a baby born through meconium-stained liquor

If a baby born through meconium-stained amniotic fluid is also floppy and makes no immediate respiratory effort, then it is reasonable to **quickly** inspect the oropharynx with a view to removing any particulate matter that might obstruct the airway. However, in a bradycardic baby the emphasis must be to inflate the lungs within the first minute after birth and this must not be delayed. There is no evidence to support routine tracheal suctioning in this situation unless there is evidence that the trachea is blocked.

> **SCREAMING BABIES HAVE AN OPEN AIRWAY**
>
> **FLOPPY BABIES – HAVE A QUICK LOOK IN THE OROPHARYNX; BUT DO NOT DELAY LUNG INFLATION**

Stiff lungs

The lungs of a sick baby at birth may sometimes be very stiff. There may have been suppression of natural surfactant production, or the lungs may have been afflicted with foreign matter such as meconium leading to decreased compliance.

In these cases, despite the manoeuvres discussed above it may not be possible to adequately inflate the lungs and oxygenate the baby. If the clinical situation suggests that stiff lungs may be a contributory factor, and you are confident that the airway is open, it may also be worth considering increasing the peak inflation pressure.

This may be sufficient to exceed the higher critical opening pressure of the stiffer lung and enable lung inflation to occur. Once inflated, the pressures required to continue with ventilatory support may be lower. Be prepared to reduce the pressures as soon as possible. There is an increased risk of air leak/pneumothorax with such stiffer lungs, especially with higher pressures.

Oxygen & monitoring

Current evidence suggests that air is sufficient in the majority of resuscitations. Where blended gas is available it is recommended that the blender be set to 21% at first. If resuscitation is prolonged, or there is a failure of the heart rate to respond to successful lung inflation then consider increasing the inspired oxygen concentration. [17, 18]

Oxygen saturation monitoring permits an estimation of the heart rate of the baby and, once stable, an indication of the level of oxygenation. Their use should be considered if the baby does not respond to initial steps.

Outside labour ward most newborn resuscitations are performed using self-inflating bags. If oxygen is available it is possible to increase the inspired oxygen to different levels (approximately 70% without using a reservoir bag [159, 160] and nearly 100% if a reservoir bag is used [161]). If oxygen is not available continue ventilating with air.

Other possible approaches

The approaches described above will allow maintenance of the airway, inflation of the lungs and support of breathing in most situations. In prolonged resuscitations or other circumstances you may consider a 'formal' airway such as a laryngeal mask airway or tracheal tube.

Laryngeal mask airway (LMA)

A laryngeal mask airway (LMA) is a supraglottic airway device, which is widely used by paediatric anaesthetists and is sometimes used in delivery suite resuscitation. [162] It can be useful in managing the difficult airway when mask ventilation fails or if tracheal intubation is difficult. The technique of inserting the LMA (and the similar i-gel) is described in Appendix 2.

There is some evidence to suggest that in infants with a gestational age of 34 weeks or above, trained practitioners may achieve successful ventilation more quickly using a LMA compared to bag valve mask ventilation. [163-165] There has been no comparison with T-piece mask ventilation and there is little experience or data on efficacy in extremely preterm infants.

Nasopharyngeal airway (NPA)

Newborn babies are nasal breathers. If the nasal airway is compromised, they may struggle. The nasopharyngeal airway (NPA) works by splinting the airway from the nostril to the pharynx. It helps in situations where the upper airway is compromised as a result of functional obstruction of the nasal passages or posterior nasal space. A typical condition where this may arise is Pierre Robin sequence – where the small jaw and abnormally shaped tongue – coupled to a cleft palate lead to restriction of the posterior nasal space.

Nasopharyngeal airways are simply flexible tubes which can be passed through the nostril and down past the tongue into the pharynx thus holding the airway open. Whilst there are specifically manufactured tubes for this purpose, a tracheal tube will suffice – ideally thin walled to increase the effective internal diameter. The technique of choosing the correct size of and inserting the NPA is described in Appendix 2.

Intubation

There are few situations in which a baby **must** be intubated. However, intubation may be indicated for the further management of respiratory distress, prolonged resuscitation, upper airway abnormalities, prolonged apnoea, diaphragmatic hernia or to provide tracheal suctioning. The technique is beyond this course and cannot be learnt from a book but the technique is described in Appendix 2.

Situations with minimal equipment

There are rare occasions when birth occurs in a setting where there is minimal or no equipment; in these situations mouth-to-mask or mouth-to-mouth resuscitation can be used.

Mouth-to-mask resuscitation

If you happen to have an appropriately sized mask and no other equipment then mouth-to-mask resuscitation is also very effective. It allows you to apply two-handed jaw thrust while at the same time holding the mask in place before applying your mouth to the mask. The pocket mask is designed for use in this way with older children and adults.

Mouth to mouth resuscitation

Mouth-to-mouth resuscitation is safe and it works. In larger babies mouth to nose resuscitation may be easier. [166] Of course, there are the usual concerns regarding transmission of potentially serious infection either to or from the baby; so use of appropriate equipment is always preferable. However, if equipment is not available it is certainly possible to resuscitate a baby at birth using this technique.

Having dried and covered the baby just remember to:

- keep the upper airway open using head position and perhaps jaw thrust, as described earlier

- cover the baby's mouth and nose with your mouth (or close the baby's mouth and use the nose alone). [166] Start with five long inflation breaths

- watch for chest movement and allow a little time for the lungs to empty before inflating the chest again. Once you have succeeded in inflating the chest shorter breaths at a rate of 20-30 breaths min^{-1} are sufficient.

Summary learning

When attempting lung aeration...

- **if the heart rate remains slow, and the chest does not move then the AIRWAY is the problem.**

- **When more common causes of failing to achieve lung aeration (incorrect head positioning, face mask leak, profound hypotonia, etc.,) have been ruled out consider tracheal obstruction even in the absence of meconium.**

If the heart rate does not improve after five inflation breaths think:

- **Is the baby's head in the neutral position?**

- **Do you need jaw thrust?**

- **Are you using a 2–3 second inflation time?**

- **Do you need a second person's help with the airway?**

- **Is there an obstruction in the oropharynx (laryngoscopy & suction)?**

- **What about an oropharyngeal airway?**

My key take-home messages from this chapter

NLS

Circulation and drugs

Contents

- **Chest compressions: when to start, technique to ensure effective compressions, ratio of breaths to compressions, length of time to perform compressions before re-assessing**
- **Drugs - when to use, which to use and route of administration**

Learning outcomes

To enable you to:

- **Consider when and why chest compressions and drugs are required in newborn resuscitation**
- **Demonstrate the techniques involved in delivering chest compressions**
- **Describe which drugs might be used, when they might be used, in what dose, and by what route they can be given**

Introduction

This chapter aims to provide an understanding of the less frequently required aspects of resuscitation in the newborn infant; namely chest compressions and drugs. It covers some of the important practical aspects. This chapter begins with chest compression (circulation), and then follows with drugs, as this is the order in which they are found in the algorithm.

Chest compressions

If airway opening manoeuvres are successful (A) and adequate lung inflation and ventilation is obtained (B), the need for chest compressions (C) lessens. [13] About 0.1% of term or near-term infants are estimated to require chest compression. [1] This percentage rises to between 2 and 10% of preterm infants. [167-169]

When are chest compressions needed?

The pulmonary circulation can be assumed to be at a standstill if the heart rate is absent or very slow (less than 60 min^{-1}) and fails to accelerate once the lungs are aerated at birth. [18] The cardiac impulse may or may not be audible or palpable, but there will be no pulsation present in the umbilical stump, skin circulation will be at a standstill, the blood pressure will be extremely low, and an ECG (if available) will probably show severe bradycardia – so called "pulseless electrical activity". Having established an airway and ensured that the chest is moving with adequate ventilation for 30 s, if the heart rate is absent or remains very slow (less than 60 min^{-1}), it is logical at this point to provide chest compressions to help get the circulation going. As ventilation is the most effective action in neonatal resuscitation and because chest compressions are likely to compete with effective ventilation, rescuers must ensure that assisted ventilation is being delivered optimally before starting chest compressions. The importance of this cannot be overstated. The only way to be sure of this is to see the chest move with each breath. The baby who does not respond to lung inflation at birth is very rare [1] and the most likely reason for failure of the heart rate to increase after attempts at lung inflation is that you have not succeeded in aerating the lungs. If using a mask check that:

- the head is in the neutral position and that the jaw is being drawn forward appropriately

- you have the right size mask and that there is a good seal against the baby's face

- there is an appropriate flow of gas to your T-piece (or that your self-inflating bag is working correctly (Chapter 6))

- you have given inflations breaths and are ventilating effectively.

> ## ABOVE ALL CHECK THAT THE CHEST IS MOVING IN RESPONSE TO YOUR VENTILATION BREATHS.

The history of chest compressions

It was in 1874, that physiological studies first showed that directly squeezing the heart, in this case of a dog, could produce a cardiac output ('open chest cardiac massage'). [170, 171] Shortly thereafter, it was also demonstrated that a similar effect could be produced by pressing on the sternum and the ribs without having to open the chest ('closed chest cardiac massage'), [172] and the successful use of such a technique in a human is attributed to Friedrich Maass in 1892. [173] Unfortunately this technique was then forgotten for over 70 years before being "accidentally rediscovered" during physiological investigations into the effects of defibrillation when Guy Knickerbocker noticed by chance that when he pressed electrode paddles firmly on the chest he could produce a rise in arterial pressure. This led to the rediscovery and reintroduction of chest compression to adult patient care as described in 1960 by William Kouwenhoven. [98]

At about the same time, interest was also being shown in the use of cardiac compressions during newborn resuscitation, [174] and a number of reports of both 'open' [175] and 'closed' [99, 176-179] cardiac massage were published in the early 1960s. Not long afterwards 'closed' massage, today known as chest compression, was being widely adopted. [178] The authors of early reports of closed chest compressions would probably recognise the techniques used today, albeit with some minor changes.

Because chest compressions are an infrequent event in newborn resuscitation there is very little scientific evidence behind the current recommendations for chest compressions in this situation. Most of the recommendations are extrapolations from animal, paediatric, and adult literature, as well as simple physiological plausibility and some expert opinion.

How do chest compressions work?

Although it was originally thought that the heart alone was emptied of blood during chest compression, it is now considered more likely that compression of the entire thorax is equally important. During the compression phase, blood is squeezed from the chest by the increased pressure in the thoracic cavity. The blood flows forward into the arteries rather than into the veins due to the venous valves at the thoracic inlet and because muscular walls keep the lumen of arteries patent whereas the thin walled veins collapse. It is important that there is enough time in the relaxation phase to allow the chest to refill with blood. [180] The cartilaginous rib cage of the newborn and the larger size of the heart relative to the chest make chest compression much easier as well as more efficient.

What am I trying to achieve?

Resuscitating babies at birth is different from resuscitating adults. In adult resuscitation you are usually dealing with a primary cardiac arrest and you need to keep oxygenated blood flowing to the brain and heart until the problem (e.g. arrhythmia, myocardial infarction) can be rectified. In the newborn baby you have a healthy heart which has been pushed beyond normal physiological limits. You are merely trying to re-establish effective heart pumping, which should happen as soon as oxygenated blood reaches it; you can usually expect it to function virtually normally thereafter. This is important because even the best performed chest compressions can achieve only a fraction (approximately one third) of the cardiac output that is seen from a spontaneously and normally beating heart. [181, 182] However preferential perfusion of the heart and brain in the hypoxic baby (Chapter 4) can improve the blood flow to these organs to approximately 50% of that seen in normal sinus rhythm provided effective resuscitation techniques are used. [183] If starting chest compressions, the inspired oxygen concentration should be increased unless this has already occurred. This supplemental oxygen should be weaned appropriately as soon as the heart rate has recovered.

Optimal method of chest compressions (two-thumb vs. two-finger technique)

Two methods [184] for performing chest compressions in newborn infants have been described and widely used; the two-thumb technique utilises the two thumbs to depress the sternum while the hands encircle the chest and the fingers provide firm support behind the back (Figure 7.1). The two-finger technique utilizes the tips of the middle and index fingers to depress the sternum, while the free hand is used to provide a firm support behind the baby's back (Figure 7.2). This latter aspect of the two-finger technique may not always be possible in a one-person resuscitation scenario.

Studies suggest that the two-thumb method is superior to the two-finger method; the two-thumb method with lateral chest wall compression (due to the encirclement of the chest) provided significantly higher mean, systolic, and diastolic blood pressures than the two-finger method. [185-188] In addition, providers using the two-thumb technique were more likely to provide compressions of the appropriate depth on manikins [189, 190] and to do so more consistently [190]. The temporary use of the two-finger technique may be more appropriate in some circumstances of single practitioner or in multiple practitioner situations when umbilical lines are being inserted. In these cases the two-thumb technique should be adopted as soon as possible.

Where should I press?

Compress the sternum over its lower third. [191-193] If you press too high on the sternum the heart is not compressed; if you press too low, you risk damaging the liver. Place your thumbs on the sternum **just** below an imaginary line joining the nipples (Figure 7.1). Do **not**, as was formerly advocated, place your thumbs one finger's breadth below this line as this can result in pressure being exerted on the xiphisternum or even the abdomen. [194]

The two-thumb (two-handed) technique

Grip the chest in both hands placing the thumbs together at the front with the fingers over the spine (Figure 7.1). Your thumbs should be on the sternum and not on the ribs on either side. [179, 185, 185, 188] In performing the two-thumb technique, overlapping the thumbs rather than placing them side-by-side provides better intrathoracic pressures for longer. [195, 196]

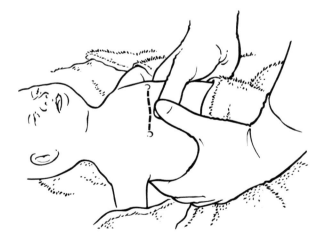

Figure 7.1 Two-thumb (two hand) chest compression

The two-finger technique

If your hands are too small to encircle the chest then a less effective alternative [185, 188] to the above method is to press at the same point on the sternum with two fingers while the back of the baby is well supported (Figure 7.2).

This may be the only method available in cases of a single person operator as one hand is used to maintain the airway. This may be useful temporarily when venous access is being obtained so that the view of the umbilical cord is not obscured.

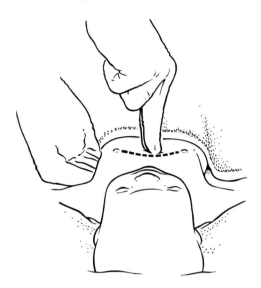

Figure 7.2 Two-finger chest compression

How deep should I press?

Compress the lower third of the sternum regularly by about one third of the depth of the chest, towards the backbone. [191, 197] There continues to be an absence of specific data about ideal compression depth and it is important to realise that although the consensus opinion was that one third of the depth of the chest would be appropriate, the depth should be adequate to produce a palpable pulse. Data from slightly older infants (median age one month) undergoing cardiac surgery suggests a depth of one half of the depth of the chest may be necessary, [198] however mathematical modelling based on chest CT scans supports that this may over-compress the heart in a significant proportion of babies. [197] What is clear from the same study is that a depth of less than one third is inadequate. Chest compression in the newborn does not cause rib fractures unless the baby has a rare severe bone disease such as osteogenesis imperfecta [199] and even then it is not an inevitable consequence. [200]

How fast should I press?

Both the compression and the recoil are important. You are not trying to reproduce a normal neonatal heart rate of about 140 min⁻¹. If you try to do so you will not produce effective blood flow because this technique is not as mechanically efficient as normal cardiac function. The rate you achieve is influenced by the chest wall compliance of the baby. Allow time after each compression for the chest to refill, by allowing it to re-expand fully. A compression to relaxation ratio with a slightly longer relaxation than compression phase offers theoretical advantages for blood flow in the very young infant. [201] Remember, you are only trying to move oxygenated blood a short distance to restart the heart.

The current guidelines recommend synchronised compressions and ventilations in a ratio of 3:1 to achieve 90 compressions and 30 breaths (i.e. 120 events) in one minute. [17, 18] In practice this can be difficult to sustain. [202] In prolonged resuscitations that extend beyond one - two minutes of cardiac compressions consideration should be given to switching personnel to prevent fatigue which may reduce the effectiveness of the compressions. [203]

Compelling animal data from adult ventricular fibrillation (VF) models indicate that frequent and prolonged interruption of chest compressions worsens coronary perfusion pressure and increases mortality. [183, 204] The situation is different in the newborn infant where lack of oxygen, rather than a cardiac dysrhythmia, leads to the arrest; in adults who have just arrested the oxygen, carbon dioxide and pH of blood is essentially normal whereas the newborn infant who has reached the stage of requiring chest compressions will be hypoxic, hypercarbic and acidotic. Thus in an adult who is in the early stages of arrest chest compressions will result in the circulation of oxygen, whereas in the baby who has reached the stage of cardiac standstill performing chest compressions without addressing the airway and breathing will simply result in the circulation of deoxygenated blood. [205-209]

In newborn babies chest compressions are delivered in a ratio of three compressions to one ventilation (3:1 ratio). This ratio is largely a consensus opinion, based on physiological plausibility but evidence is emerging to support its use. In one study using manikins, a greater depth of compression was achieved, and operators were more likely to sustain the correct depth for longer, when using a 3:1 versus 15:2 ratio. [210] The minute ventilation is greater when using a 3:1 versus 15:2 ratio [211] and in a porcine model of newborn hypoxia other ratios (e.g. 9:3 and 15:2) appeared to offer no advantage in terms of time to the return of spontaneous circulation or other post-resuscitation parameters. [212, 213]

If during resuscitation the baby has a tracheal tube placed, intermittent compressions and ventilations are continued using the same 3:1 ratio. Continuous, asynchronised, chest compressions are used in adults particularly when intubated but are **not** recommended in newborns. In a porcine model of newborn hypoxia where the animal was intubated with a cuffed tracheal tube (thus minimising any leak) asynchronous compressions did not result in an earlier return of spontaneous circulation than the currently recommended 3:1 ratio. [214] The potential for asynchronous compressions to interfere with ventilation was reflected in almost a third of breaths being affected by compressions and that blood gas parameters after the return of spontaneous circulation were worse than in the 3:1 group. Little is known about how asynchronous compressions would impact on breaths in the non-intubated baby receiving mask ventilation.

How long should I continue?

One would expect the heart rate to respond quickly to effective chest compressions, usually within 20–30 s. [13] Recheck the heart rate every 30 s to detect any response.

What if I get no response?

If you get no response to adequate chest compression combined with effective lung inflation and ventilation, the most likely reasons are myocardial dysfunction secondary to lactic acidosis, pulseless electrical activity (formerly known as "electro-mechanical dissociation") or possibly exhaustion of myocardial glycogen. You will now need to consider using drugs.

When are drugs needed?

Drugs should only be considered if, despite aerating the lungs, the circulation has failed and the heart does not respond to effective ventilation and good quality chest compressions. This is a very rare event, occurring in less than 1 in 2000 deliveries in one large series of nearly 38,000 deliveries. [1] Although drugs have been used in this situation for decades there is very little human evidence that they are effective and, though some babies appear to respond initially, the outlook is generally very poor. [215] Some studies report better results but careful reading suggests that drugs were sometimes used before the airway had been attended to and therefore these drugs were presumably given unnecessarily. [169, 216]

The most likely reason for chest compression failing to achieve a response is that it has been started before the lungs have been effectively aerated. Before using drugs check that the chest is definitely moving in response to inflation (and then the on-going ventilation) breaths either delivered by mask or tracheal tube and that the chest compressions are being performed appropriately.

> **DRUGS ARE USELESS WITHOUT EFFECTIVE VENTILATION**

How should drugs be given?

In the baby who requires drugs, the circulation is not functioning and so drugs must be delivered as close as possible to the heart. This is best achieved by using an umbilical venous catheter (UVC). The technique for insertion of a UVC is described in Appendix 2. Injections into a peripheral vein are unlikely to reach the heart when there is complete circulatory arrest, even with good quality basic life support that includes chest compressions. Direct injections into the umbilical cord vessels are useless for the same reason. One very significant reason for avoiding peripheral lines is that umbilical catheterisation is much quicker and easier in the baby whose peripheral circulation has 'shut down'.

Catheterisation of the umbilical vein to provide venous access for an exchange transfusion in cases of Rhesus disease was first reported in 1946. [217] Since then they have been used to provide central access in sick babies for a variety of reasons including administration of inotropes, parenteral nutrition [218] or hypertonic solutions, angiography, [219] and blood sampling. The first published report of use during resuscitation did not appear until 1980. [220]

An alternative to the umbilical venous route is the intraosseus route [221] (Appendix 2) which is more frequently used to provide emergency central venous access in older infants and children. In simulated newborn resuscitations they can be inserted as quickly as an umbilical venous catheter. [222, 223] The intraosseus route may also be useful in the very rare situation when a baby who has an abnormal umbilical cord and who also needs drugs during resuscitation. [224]

Adrenaline may be given by the tracheal route provided the baby is intubated[225] but cannot be recommended as there are serious doubts as to whether it is effective in the newborn. If it is to have any effect it is likely that the dose required is significantly higher than that used intravenously. [226, 227] None of the other drugs mentioned below can be given this way.

DRUGS SHOULD BE GIVEN CENTRALLY

What drugs should I use?

Adrenaline (epinephrine = rINN)

- **Preparation** 1:10,000 (= 1 g/10,000 mL = 100 mg/L = 100 microgram/mL)

- **Dose** 10 microgram kg^{-1} (0.1 mL kg^{-1} of 1:10,000)

- **Route** Umbilical venous catheter or intra-osseous needle (may be given via a tracheal tube but see the caveats below)

Animal evidence suggests that adrenaline cannot bind to its receptors at very low pH. [226] If there is no response to a dose of 10 microgram kg^{-1} it is arguably worth giving a dose of bicarbonate (see below) and then a further larger dose of adrenaline of 30 microgram kg^{-1} (i.e. 0.3 mL kg of a 1:10,000 solution).

Unlike the other drugs mentioned in this section, adrenaline can be safely given down a tracheal tube. [227] However, if a standard 10–30 microgram kg^{-1} dose is given by this route it is not likely to be effective. A higher dose of at least 50 microgram kg^{-1} (maximum 100 microgram kg^{-1}) by this route might be considered but the safety and efficacy of such a dose has not been determined and is not recommended unless there is no other option. Use of standard doses via the umbilical venous or intraosseus route is preferred (see Appendix 1).

In cardiac arrest, adrenaline acts via alpha-adrenergic receptor-mediated vasoconstriction [228, 229] to elevate the aortic to right atrial pressure gradient during the relaxation phase of cardiopulmonary resuscitation. [230] This increases coronary artery perfusion pressure, which in cardiac arrest due to abnormal rhythms is directly related to both myocardial blood flow and return of spontaneous circulation. [231]

The evidence for the most appropriate dose of adrenaline in any age group is sadly lacking; the initial animal studies of adrenaline used an arbitrary dose of 1 mg (which approximated to about 0.1 mg kg^{-1} for the average dogs used in the studies). [228, 232] The same 1 mg dose was then adopted in humans without any adjustments for the bigger size of the typical adult – this resulted in an approximate weight-based dose of 10 microgram kg^{-1}. This dose was subsequently adopted in paediatric and neonatal protocols despite the lack of evidence behind it.

Adult and paediatric protocols started to recommend increasing the dose of adrenaline ten-fold (0.1 mg kg^{-1}) if there was no initial response to 0.01 mg kg^{-1} when evidence from animal studies suggested that high-doses improved blood flow to the brain and heart, [233] as well as the return of spontaneous circulation. [234] The high doses were not adopted in newborn resuscitation for a variety of reasons; a multi-centre, randomised, double-blind trial of high (100 microgram kg^{-1}) versus standard dose adrenaline (10 microgram kg^{-1}) in children found a lower 24 hour survival for the high-dose group especially in those children whose arrest was secondary to hypoxia. [235] In a randomised, blinded trial of high versus standard dose adrenaline in neonatal piglets subjected to acute severe hypoxia there was no advantage in terms of survival at 24 hours, but high doses caused tachycardia and hypertension. [236] This period of hypertension, immediately after the hypotension that occurs during cardiac arrest increases the risk of intraventricular haemorrhage. [237]

Glucose

- **Preparation** 10% (= 10g/100 mL = 100mg/mL)

- **Dose** 250 mg kg^{-1} (2.5 mL kg^{-1} of 10%)

- **Route** Umbilical venous catheter or intra-osseous needle

The heart cannot work without glucose and the glycogen stores present in the heart at birth are rapidly depleted during prolonged hypoxia. Glucose can be tried if there is no response to adrenaline and bicarbonate. 10% glucose is quite concentrated enough to supply a bolus of fuel to the heart.

Subsequent symptomatic hypoglycaemia, if present, is better managed with an infusion of 10% glucose rather than with repeated boluses. Glucose must never be given down the tracheal tube.

During hypoxia, anaerobic metabolism and glycolysis rapidly depletes hepatic glycogen and glucose production rapidly becomes insufficient to meet cerebral metabolic demand. The evidence for the use of glucose in this situation is poor. Studies have shown a significant positive linear correlation between plasma glucose level and Apgar scores, and a significant negative linear correlation between the glucose level and severity of stages of hypoxic ischemic encephalopathy (HIE). [238] Indirect evidence from infants with hypoxic ischaemic encephalopathy shows early hypoglycaemia (up to six hours of age) was associated with a more severe HIE, and adverse neurological outcome. [239, 240]

Administration of glucose might therefore be seen as logical in prolonged resuscitation, and has been recommended in unresponsive newborn bradycardia or asystole. However, there is no human evidence that administering glucose improves outcomes and the animal data are conflicting as to its effect on neurological outcomes.

Sodium bicarbonate

- **Preparation**   4.2% (or 8.4% diluted 1:1 with 5% or 10% Glucose)

- **Dose**   1–2 mmol kg^{-1} (2–4 mL kg^{-1} of 4.2%)

- **Route**   Umbilical venous catheter or intra-osseous needle

NOTE: 1 mL of 8.4% sodium bicarbonate contains 1 mmol

If there is no effective cardiac output, or virtually none, then reversing intracardiac acidosis may be helpful. This is certainly true in animal experiments. [79] You are not attempting to correct the baby's metabolic acidosis; you are merely trying to improve cardiac function by improving the pH of the blood within the heart.

An alkalising agent will normally produce cardiac acceleration within a couple of minutes if it is going to work. Bicarbonate must **never** be given down the tracheal tube.

Volume

- **Preparation**   0.9% saline, (or a balanced salt solution)

- **Dose**   10 mL kg^{-1} initially

- **Route**   Umbilical venous catheter or intra-osseous needle

A bolus of about 10 mL kg^{-1} is usually sufficient to produce a response and can be repeated if necessary. If blood loss is the cause of the problem further transfusion with blood may be necessary later. Giving further volume to a severely compromised baby with a myocardium damaged by hypoxia is likely to do more harm than good.

Giving large volumes (more than 40 mL kg^{-1}) of solutions high in chloride (such as albumin or 0.9% saline) can also exacerbate metabolic acidosis through hyperchloraemia. [241]

After each of the drugs has been given use a small flush of 0.9% sodium chloride to ensure the drug reaches the circulation and a few chest compressions to ensure the drug then reaches the heart, and then assess the effect.

Summary learning

- **Use chest compressions when there is a very slow (<60 min^{-1}) or absent heart beat and you are sure that you have inflated the lungs.**

- **Press down quickly and firmly and then release.**

- **Aim to reduce the antero-posterior diameter of the chest by about one third with each compression.**

- **Pause after each release to allow the chest to recoil fully.**

- **Too rapid a rate gives the chambers of the heart no chance to refill passively after compression.**

- **Ventilate the lungs after every 3 compressions.**

- **If bradycardia persists despite about 30 seconds of chest compression and adequate ventilation, insert an umbilical venous catheter and administer adrenaline and/or sodium bicarbonate, followed by further chest compressions.**

- **Glucose and volume expansion may, rarely, be needed.**

- **If lung inflation and ventilation breaths followed by chest compressions are not working then the outcome even with drugs is likely to be poor.**

My key take-home messages from this chapter

Preterm babies

Contents

- Definition of preterm and which preterm babies are different
- Delayed cord clamping
- Thermal care of the preterm baby
- Supporting pulmonary gas exchange and avoiding lung damage
- Saturation monitoring

Learning outcomes

To enable you to:

- Appreciate that most preterm babies require help with transition rather than resuscitation
- Understand how to support the transition of preterm babies
- Understand why attention to temperature is vital in these babies
- Appreciate the importance of avoiding harm caused by hypothermia, hyperoxia, hyperventilation by using pulse oximetry to guide oxygen use, CPAP or, if required, gentle ventilation (lower inflation pressures, PEEP and prophylactic surfactant)

Degrees of prematurity

Epidemiologically speaking, term babies are those born between 37 completed weeks of gestation and 42 weeks but the way this definition was arrived at can hardly be described as a triumph of the scientific method. [122] There are exceptions to every rule but, based purely on gestation, the probability of a baby needing significant assistance at delivery if born between 34 and 37 weeks gestation is little different from that of more mature babies. However, at 30 weeks gestation and below it is a different matter and every effort should be made to ensure that a senior person with extensive experience in dealing with preterm babies is present at their delivery (Figure 8.1).

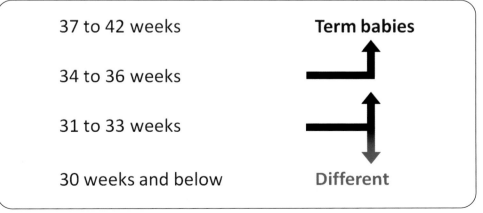

37 to 42 weeks	**Term babies**
34 to 36 weeks	
31 to 33 weeks	
30 weeks and below	**Different**

Figure 8.1 Using gestation to guide the approach to resuscitation

NLS

Effective teamwork and communication within the team and the neonatal unit is essential if these vulnerable babies are not to be exposed to, what is for them, a cold and hostile environment for any longer than is necessary. The remainder of this chapter is primarily concerned with these babies.

Assisting transition rather than resuscitation

Most preterm babies are in reasonable condition at birth and are only in need of assisted transition, not resuscitation. [242] In other words they are fragile individuals needing careful handling and gentle support, not critically ill babies on the point of death. Provided babies can be kept warm it is to their advantage that clamping of the cord is delayed and they remain attached to the placenta for a period while establishing pulmonary respiration. [243]

Allow delayed cord clamping to occur

The benefits (Table 8.1) of delayed cord clamping in preterm infants are more firmly established than for term babies. [244, 245]

- Increased circulating blood volume after birth
- Improved cardiovascular stability
- Decreased need for blood transfusion
- Decreased risk of intraventricular haemorhage
- Decreased risk of necrotising enterocolitis

Table 8.1 The benefits of delayed cord clamping in preterm infants

Provided you can maintain the baby's temperature and the baby does not need immediate resuscitation, delayed cord clamping should be performed in all preterm deliveries where the placenta is still attached to the uterus to allow placental transfusion. This approach requires communication and teamwork by all midwifery, obstetric and paediatric staff involved.

Delayed cord clamping helps to maintain venous return to the heart while the blood vessels in the lungs are filled. Recent studies in a sheep model of fetal to neonatal transition have shown that delaying cord clamping **after** the initiation of positive pressure ventilation and establishment of a functional residual capacity (resting lung volume) results in increased myocardial stability, carotid flow, and brain oxygenation and makes the transition process smoother. [68]

There remains some equipoise surrounding the length of time to delay cord clamping, and studies have looked at delays between 30 s and 430 s. Local policy should be referred to regarding length of time for delayed cord clamping in your hospital. The baby can be assessed during this time.

There is insufficient evidence to advise on the optimal position of the baby during delayed cord clamping. [246] One randomised trial showed that position of the baby during delayed cord clamping (at level of introitus or on maternal chest) made no difference to the volume of placental transfusion, however this study was in term newborns. [247] The pragmatic approach is to place the baby between mother's legs, or on her abdomen or chest, during delayed cord clamping and to avoid having the baby at a level where gravity may have an adverse effect on placental transfer.

Whilst delayed cord clamping is the preferred choice, where the condition of the baby is assessed as being in need of immediate assistance, cord milking **may** be considered using the techniques described in randomised trials published to date. [248] This manoeuvre consists of clamping the cord near the placenta and milking approximately 20 cm three times from the placenta end of the cord towards the baby. This can be performed in a few seconds; it provides the baby with an additional volume of blood and should not unduly delay any resuscitation. Whilst several short-term benefits have been described, the long-term benefits have not; thus cord milking should only be considered on an individualised basis (or as part of a well-designed randomised controlled trial). [249]

Once the cord is cut, the baby should be promptly taken to a resuscitaire in a polythene bag and standard warming measures as discussed below should be employed.

Keeping the baby warm – polythene bags and radiant heat

Why?

The preterm infant is particularly vulnerable to heat loss and subsequent hypothermia, as they have immature thin skin, reduced subcutaneous fat, poor vasomotor control and an increased body surface to mass ratio.

There is an increased mortality associated with hypothermia especially in small and preterm babies, and for every 1°C below 36.5°C the risk of mortality increases by up to 28%. [32, 33]. Mortality is highest at lower admission temperatures and admission temperatures less than 32.9°C have been associated with more than 80% mortality. [250] Even a brief period of hypothermia is associated with neonatal morbidity; impaired surfactant synthesis, impaired surfactant spreading within the lungs, pulmonary hypertension, hypoxia and coagulation defects. Acidosis and hypoxia further inhibit surfactant production. [26, 251]

Hypothermia may be a marker for increased risk of death, especially in infants who continue to lose heat during stabilisation. Meticulous attention to temperature remains an integral part of the approach to the preterm infant at delivery.

How?

Environmental temperature: Raise the delivery room or operating theatre temperature, ideally to at least 26°C for babies less than 28 weeks gestation. [38, 252]

Polythene bags under radiant heat: There is now good evidence that it is easier to maintain the temperature of very preterm babies if they are placed immediately after birth, without drying, into a polythene bag. [253, 254] It is important to remember that the babies in these studies were also then placed under a radiant heater.

Some specially designed bags are available but any bags approved for use for wrapping food when cooked in a microwave may also be used. Obviously the face should not be covered with polythene but it is helpful to cover the baby's head with a hat. If you need access to areas of the baby within the polythene bag, a small cut can be made in the bag for this purpose. Once the baby is on the resuscitaire do not cover the polythene bag with anything else but leave directly under the radiant heater.

Polythene bags without radiant heat: Presumably the main advantage of using a polythene bag is that it substantially reduces evaporation of liquid from the surface of the baby. Wrapping a baby in polythene and then placing the baby next to a warm object – such as its mother's skin – and covering both with a warm towel will probably keep the baby warmer than a similar baby not covered in polythene but the data is not available to prove this. This strategy could be employed for preterm babies delivered outside hospital, as a means to keep them warm whilst en route to a hospital. [255, 256]

Helping to establish pulmonary gas exchange

The lungs are fragile: The lungs of preterm infants are more fragile and less compliant than those of term infants. At the same time the chest wall of the preterm infant is more compliant and less able to protect the lung against over-inflation. Over-enthusiastic inflation of fragile lungs can predispose to serious inflammatory damage and long-term morbidity. [257, 258]

CPAP & PEEP from birth: If the baby is breathing spontaneously then applying continuous positive airway pressure (CPAP) will ease the work of breathing and help to prevent alveolar collapse in expiration. Many very preterm babies can be stabilised on CPAP at birth without any need for intubation. [119, 259] Suitable CPAP levels are five to eight cm water. In the ventilated baby, airway recruitment can be increased and end-expiratory airway collapse reduced by maintaining positive end expiratory pressure (PEEP). An appropriate starting PEEP in this circumstance is 5 cm water.

Gentle and gradual aeration: If lung expansion and positive pressure ventilation is needed at birth then the aim should be to gently expand the lungs of the infant so as to gradually maximise gas exchange surface area, to avoid over-distension while at the same time preventing collapse during expiration.

In experiments in preterm lambs use of large inflation volumes immediately after delivery caused significant damage. This damage was slightly less if surfactant was given before inflation. However, if large tidal volumes were only used after 10 min of more gentle ventilation much less damage was done. [260] This would suggest that a more gradual approach may be an advantage rather than aiming for rapid achievement of full lung inflation.

It is probably 'unreasonable' to attempt to fully inflate the lungs of the preterm infant too quickly, just as it is 'unreasonable' to expect a baby to achieve adult oxygen saturation levels immediately at birth. The fetus happily copes with its relatively hypoxic environment; its arterial partial pressure of oxygen (PaO_2) is 3.0–3.5 kPa (25–30 mmHg) and in the first few minutes after birth this will increase to 10.5–12.0 kPa (80–90 mmHg). Various researchers have now shown that brief and sudden exposure of the fetus that has existed happily with its relative hypoxia to high concentrations of inspired oxygen could well have detrimental effects. [261-263]

Tidal volume: Significant damage can be caused by a small number of over-enthusiastic breaths. We can guard against this volume trauma to some extent by limiting the pressure applied to the gas in the airway but the best way is by limiting the volume change of the lung itself. This implies that the future may lie in measuring and adjusting the tidal volume administered rather than trying to estimate this clinically or via a proxy measurement of pressure. [118]

If it is possible to include devices measuring expired tidal volume into equipment used for stabilising preterm infants at birth these may be helpful. Exactly what tidal volumes are safe and effective is not yet known but they should probably not be allowed to exceed 6–8 mL kg^{-1}, which approximates the normal tidal volume of a healthy, spontaneously breathing term infant. [264]

Pressure and volume: If you are using a T-piece, start with inflation pressures of 20–25 cm water. Even then it is still possible to inadvertently produce tidal volumes of 10 mL kg^{-1}. If these pressures, applied for a sufficient inspiratory time, are unsuccessful higher pressures can be tried. Sustained pressures of up to 30 cm water may be required [127, 180] but should be avoided if possible to reduce the risk of lung injury in survivors.

The best guide as to whether satisfactory lung inflation is being maintained is a sustained increase in the heart rate. If the heart rate has increased satisfactorily then ventilation is probably adequate. Only if the heart rate has not stabilised should you seek to increase the degree of chest expansion. Clinical judgement is unreliable when assessing tidal volume based on chest excursion. [265, 266]

If significant chest expansion is easily seen it is likely that inflation volumes are too great and over-distension of the lung may be occurring.

If a preterm infant appears to need continued ventilation rather than CPAP then the baby should be connected to a modern ventilator as soon as possible and the settings adjusted to avoid excessive tidal volume.

> **Avoid over-distension of the lungs Start with pressures of 20 cm water and use PEEP (5 cm water)**

Intubation

Few preterm babies, even below 28 weeks gestation, require intubation at birth in order to survive. Some babies will also deliver unexpectedly outside the labour ward where the attendant may not only be inexperienced at intubation but may also have minimal equipment. It is safer to avoid intubation in such circumstances. [267] The normal algorithm should be followed, paying particular attention to drying the baby and keeping the baby covered and warm or placing into a polythene bag and placed next to the mother's skin, and instituting good airway control and mask ventilation if necessary.

Intubation with the correct size tube will make the ventilation of abnormally stiff lungs easier. It will also allow administration of surfactant. Inflation pressures should be delivered in a controlled manner in order to avoid excessive inspiratory volumes, which might risk significant lung injury. Control of inspiratory pressure is most easily achieved using a T-piece system rather than a bag-mask device. Ideally PEEP should be applied to reduce alveolar collapse in expiration and thus avoid the inevitable shearing forces which occur when collapsed alveoli and small airways are re-expanded. [117, 268]

Surfactant therapy: For babies less than 30 weeks gestation there is a serious risk of Respiratory Distress Syndrome (RDS) and evidence that early prophylactic use of surfactant has advantages over rescue treatment. [268, 269] Any baby of 30 weeks or less who has a tracheal tube placed should almost certainly receive surfactant; in some it may even allow early extubation and use of CPAP. Early use of surfactant and CPAP can reduce the number of preterm babies needing long-term ventilation. [268] Some units administer surfactant in the delivery room, others on the neonatal unit.

Avoid both hyperoxaemia and hypoxia

Stabilisation or resuscitation of significantly preterm babies (30 weeks or less) may be started with air or supplemental oxygen up to 30%. However, use of oxygen should be monitored using pulse oximetry.

Using a pulse oximeter to monitor both heart rate and oxygen saturation in these babies from birth makes

stabilisation much easier (Appendix 3). Exposing babies at birth to high concentrations of oxygen can have significant adverse longer term effects. [270, 271] The study reporting normal values for right arm (pre-ductal) oxygen saturation levels in the first minutes after birth from over 450 babies contained data from only 39 babies born before 32 weeks gestation. [112] The 25th centile saturation levels in these preterm babies was very slightly lower than the same centile constructed from the data from all the babies in the study. Table 8.2 is the same as that in Chapter 5 and shows the 25th centile values for **all** the babies in the study.

Time from birth	Acceptable (25th centile) right arm saturation (%)
2 min	60
3 min	70
4 min	80
5 min	85
10 min	90

Table 8.2 Acceptable right arm oxygen saturations after birth

For practical purposes the same values of 'acceptable' oxygen saturation can be used for both term and preterm infants. Remember, these saturation levels are deemed 'acceptable' in the sense that babies exhibiting these levels or higher probably do not need any supplemental oxygen. However, babies whose saturation levels are significantly lower might warrant careful supplementation.

And the rare preterm baby who actually needs resuscitation?

Rapid and accurate assessment of the condition of a preterm baby at birth requires some experience but, just as in term infants, preterm babies delivered in poor condition due to hypoxia or hypovolaemia require prompt resuscitation. If the baby does not have an effective circulation or if there has been placental abruption then there is unlikely to be any advantage in delaying clamping the umbilical cord.

Warmth: These infants should be placed in a polythene bag under a radiant heater immediately and be resuscitated as judged necessary using the standard approach to airway, breathing and circulation. The presence of hypoxia adds urgency to the need to establish effective ventilation and the situation is no longer one of encouraging gentle transition. Any hypoxia will continue until effective aeration and ventilation is established.

Lower inflation pressures: Start with five inflation breaths at pressures of 20–25 cm water with a background PEEP of five cm water. Then check the heart rate and, if the heart rate is not improving, ventilation pressures should be increased until visible chest expansion is identifiable.

Consider reducing ventilation pressures as soon as you achieve a response.

Although preterm infants at risk of RDS may benefit from surfactant replacement, this should not be considered a drug of resuscitation as a bolus of surfactant may briefly compromise ventilation before it becomes more widely distributed.

Summary learning

- Most preterm babies need support and 'assisted transition' in the minutes after birth rather than resuscitation.

- Clamping of the cord should be delayed unless exceptional circumstances.

- Polythene bags and overhead warming are the best methods for preventing hypothermia.

- Establish oxygen saturation monitoring as soon as you can and adjust the air/oxygen blender to avoid hyperoxia and hypoxia.

- If the baby has satisfactory oxygen saturation and heart rate and is making regular breathing attempts try mask CPAP, starting with air.

- If the baby does not breathe, begin with inflation breaths at 20–25 cm water, starting with air.

- If the preterm baby does need intubating, consider early use of surfactant.

My key take-home messages from this chapter

Birth outside labour ward

Contents

- **Planned homebirths**
- **Environment**
- **Personnel at birth**
- **Management of the 3rd stage of labour**
- **Calling for help**
- **Transfer to hospital**
- **Birth in an ambulance**
- **Record keeping**

Learning outcomes

To enable you to:

- **Understand the practitioner's role in preparing to manage effective resuscitation of the newborn baby in planned or unplanned birth outside the hospital labour ward**
- **Prepare equipment, environment and junior colleagues to support effective resuscitation of the newborn**
- **Balance the psychological needs of the mother and family, with ensuring the safety of mother and baby through birth and early postnatal period**
- **Appreciate the key issues to be included in record keeping around resuscitation of the newborn**

Introduction

Birth outside labour ward may be planned or unplanned. Planned home births usually involve low risk pregnancies in which the birth is *"due to take place after 37 completed weeks to 42 weeks gestation and a normal birth is expected"*. [272]

For planned home births, the woman, her partner and all healthcare individuals can collaborate and agree details concerning who will attend the birth, when and how they will be called, what equipment will be needed, how it will be obtained, and what the backup arrangements are in case of emergencies. However, if the birth is unplanned, none of these arrangements will have been made; in addition the pregnancy may not be a "low risk" pregnancy for either the mother or the baby. It may further be complicated by the baby being preterm. [273] This chapter will aim to cover both situations with suggestions as to how to resuscitate the baby as safely and effectively as possible.

In the majority of situations where birth occurs outside hospital, the professional supervising the birth is a midwife. The midwife's duty is to provide care to both woman and baby. While resuscitating the baby the midwife must be aware of the physical and psychological well-being of the mother and at no time while resuscitating the baby should the mother be out of the vision and hearing of the midwife.

Government policy in all four countries of the UK is to promote choice for women in relation to their pregnancy care and place of birth, and these should include a range of birth environments to meet the needs of mothers and their babies. [274-276] This has resulted in increased numbers of births outside acute hospitals. A number of official documents have been drawn up, by government and professional bodies, relating to and regulating this process. [277, 278]

Planned home births

Planned births outside hospital should be only be offered when there are clear and timely referral and transfer arrangements in place in case of emergencies or complications. The suitability of home births should be discussed in advance with the woman and her partner. In a woman who is 'low risk' in their second and subsequent pregnancies, a planned home birth is as safe as hospital birth for the baby, and less likely to involve medical intervention to the mother. [279]

Commissioners and providers of maternity care should ensure that there are:

- robust protocols in place for transfer of care between settings

- clear local pathways for the continued care of women who are transferred from one setting to another.

Furthermore in some localities this should also take into consideration the need to cross provider boundaries if the nearest obstetric or neonatal unit is closed to admissions or the local midwifery-led unit is full.

All NHS maternity care providers must ensure that community based facilities are 'fully equipped and staff have the skills for initial management and referral of obstetric and neonatal emergencies'. During the antenatal period the woman and her family should have been made aware of the on-call arrangements, the preparations to be made within the home, what equipment may be required and any transfer arrangements and procedures.

Although the recommendations for the initial management of the baby born through meconium stained liquor no longer require routine intubation of the apnoeic baby, the significance of meconium as an indicator of fetal compromise should lead to a transfer of care to a hospital setting provided that it is safe to do so and the birth is unlikely to occur before transfer is completed.

Environment
Preparing the environment

A suitable area for attending to the baby needs to be

identified and prepared in advance. A firm, flat elevated surface area should be cleared and towels or substitutes made ready.

Close the windows and doors to prevent draughts. Use stand-alone heaters or heated mattress if available. Consider the kitchen as the area for resuscitation and use warm radiators to heat towels. But be careful not to overheat them; test the temperature against the inner aspect of your forearm. Hot water bottles can also be useful to heat the surface area but should never be put in direct contact with the baby.

Temperature

Maintaining the normal temperature of the baby can be more difficult outside hospital, but it remains equally, if not more important as in a hospital setting. Cover the baby's head with a hat and then, if appropriate, place the baby in direct skin-to-skin contact with the mother, or another warm adult body, under a dry towel or under clothing. If skin-to-skin contact is provided it is vital to observe the newborn baby's airway at all times and the woman needs to be made aware of the importance of this by, for example, avoiding other distractions such as using social media. [50, 51] Alternatively the baby should be dried and wrapped in warm towels or clothing. Polythene bags are a further option in both term and preterm babies outside of labour wards when the delivery is unplanned or the baby is ill, however a heat source will also be required. [255, 256]

Timing

Use your watch or a clock in the house, preferably one that shows seconds as well as hours and minutes, to enable accurate documentation of times.

Equipment

Exactly what equipment should be carried for planned home births is a matter for local decision. Some equipment may be provided by the family. A suggested minimum list is available through the Resuscitation Council (UK) website (www.resus.org.uk).

The choice of equipment is very much a pragmatic one, the T-piece and blender combinations that allow accurate and controlled delivery of variable pressures and variable oxygen concentrations in a hospital setting are not currently available in a form that is very suitable for a home birth as the additional weight is often prohibitive. T-piece equipment is, however, becoming more portable and may lend itself to being able to deliver variable pressure from portable cylinders, however delivering a variable oxygen concentration using the same equipment is not easy. A self-inflating bag, however, allows the delivery of inflation breaths using room air with the ability to increase the inspired oxygen to different levels; oxygen concentrations of approximately 70% can be achieved by attaching an oxygen supply to the self-inflating bag without its reservoir bag if this can be removed [160, 161] and nearly 100% if a reservoir bag is used [162].

At birth

If possible two healthcare professionals, at least one of whom should be a registered midwife, need to be present at the birth. Tasks should be allocated depending on the situation and the skills of those available.

Detailed discussion of the midwifery and obstetric practicalities are beyond the scope of this text, but physiological management of the third stage is likely to be more appropriate in this situation and will allow for delayed cord clamping. It also becomes easier to focus attention on the baby if physiological management of the third stage is used. Active management of the third stage using syntometrine may delay attendance on the baby. The resuscitation of the newborn in the home, as in any other environment, follows the standard algorithm.

Help

Within any locality where home births take place an agreed system of 'who should be called when' needs to be in place. In most cases help will be available via an emergency call for a paramedic ambulance but in more remote areas other means may be used. If the home does not have a landline or mobile phone reception then an alternative needs to be arranged.

Transfer

If a baby has needed resuscitation at birth then transfer to hospital is required following stabilisation. If only one midwife is present then both the mother and her baby should be transferred and not be separated during that transfer unless this is unavoidable. The ambulance staff should be asked to increase the temperature in the ambulance prior to transfer. If the temperature is uncomfortably warm for an adult it will be about right for the baby.

If the baby is maintaining his airway well, then he can be transported held close to mother. However, if the baby requires support then special arrangements will be needed. It is unusual for a neonatal transport team to travel to the home with a transport incubator; instead usual practice is for the baby to be brought to a hospital. If a decision has been made to bring the baby into hospital whilst still being resuscitated the stretcher is used as a base to resuscitate the baby. Insert a board or tray to level surface area of the stretcher then cover with towels and place the baby on the top to continue resuscitation procedures. The environment should be as warm as possible. Remember to consider the safety of the whole team in this situation.

Unplanned births outside labour ward

Help must be called early - you will almost certainly need it. Unplanned births are more likely to be premature or involving babies or women with health problems. An unplanned birth may occur anywhere a pregnant woman might be. The approach to resuscitation is the same anywhere but the availability of equipment, personnel and experience will obviously vary. [280]

Mouth-to-mouth resuscitation (Chapter 6) may be required if the baby is not breathing.

Birth in an ambulance

Stop the Ambulance

It is not possible to manage a birth safely in a moving ambulance. Ask the crew to stop the ambulance and increase the heating. One of the ambulance crew should make immediate radio contact with ambulance control who can relay the information to the nearest maternity unit or other centre.

Mother

Ask the mother to sit upright if possible as this will leave space to deal with the newborn. Leave the cord intact while you assess the baby and the need for resuscitation. Leave the placenta to deliver physiologically after cutting the cord. Support the mother and do not attempt to deliver the placenta in transit. Observe progress of the third stage of labour and monitor for bleeding.

Baby

The baby should be resuscitated, if needed, in the standard manner. Once the baby is safely born, make sure the baby is kept warm, continue to make clinical observations and restart the journey. A baby in good condition can be given to the mother for skin-to-skin contact (Figure 3.1), or else wrapped and held by the mother. Plastic bags can also be useful in this situation.[255, 256]

Record keeping

Clinical records of the birth at home must be maintained in exactly the same way as they are for births in a hospital setting. These records must be continued during the transfer.

Summary learning

In birth outside the hospital setting, take control of the environment and follow the same principles

- **Call for help early**

- **Dry, warm and cover the baby**

- **Assess**

- **Open the airway, use inflation breaths (air)**

- **Chest compressions if successful inflation but no response**

- **Continue until help arrives and insure appropriate handover**

**My key take-home messages
from this chapter**

Post-resuscitation care, prognostication and communication

Contents

- Immediate and later post-resuscitation monitoring and care
- Determining the likely cause for requiring resuscitation including whether a baby was probably in primary or secondary apnoea
- When to consider therapeutic hypothermia
- The prognosis of babies requiring resuscitation
- Keeping accurate records and communicating with parents and professional colleagues after a resuscitation

Learning outcomes

To enable you to:

- **Understand the need to assess risk of further physiological problems requiring stabilisation and transfer to a neonatal unit for high dependency or possibly intensive care following significant resuscitation**
- **Describe some of the most common problems which may occur after significant resuscitation**
- **Discuss the use of use of therapeutic hypothermia (cooling) for babies with hypoxic ischaemic encephalopathy (HIE); who can be treated and how and when it should be considered**
- **Understand that good communication is critically important in the support of distressed parents and the healthcare team and in avoidance of complaints and litigation**

Introduction

This chapter attempts to summarise current opinion on some of the key aspects of further management following the need for significant resuscitation at birth, including a summary of prognostic factors and the importance of good communication and record keeping. The reader should be aware that this is not a comprehensive list and the review represents current opinion as well as evidence where evidence exists. Most babies who require some resuscitation at birth will quickly stabilise and may remain with their parents, however some babies will require additional monitoring and sometimes support.

Immediate post-resuscitation care

(a) Monitoring return of circulation and breathing

Behaviour during recovery from a hypoxic insult is a guide to the length and severity of the episode and should be monitored and documented carefully. Once the circulation is restored, agonal gasping, occurring every 5–8 s, is almost always the first sign of recovery from terminal apnoea. Ventilation should continue until normal regular breathing is established. Gasping may continue after normal respiratory activity appears. One indicator of the duration and or severity of the hypoxic insult to the

NLS

central nervous system is the length of time from the return of a normal heart rate to the onset of normal regular respiration (with or without intermittent additional gasps). [76, 85]

(b) Continued airway support

If intubation has been necessary and if extubation is not appropriate, the tracheal tube must be well secured, with equal breath sounds audible on both sides of the chest, before transfer to the neonatal unit. Positive end expiratory pressure (PEEP) should be used during transfer, or at least as soon as possible on reaching the neonatal unit. Any dead space should be minimised by trimming the tracheal tube. Avoid over-ventilation during transfer and try to avoid both hyperoxaemia and hypocarbia. [281] Consider exogenous surfactant in any intubated and ventilated baby in whom surfactant-deficiency may lead to Respiratory Distress Syndrome (RDS). [282]

(c) Decisions about post-resuscitation care

Once the initial stabilisation phase is over, a care plan is needed which balances the desire to keep the baby with the mother where possible, against the need for close observation and high dependency support in babies at significant risk of post-resuscitation problems. [283]

When making decisions about post-resuscitation care, the following factors need to be incorporated in a thoughtful risk assessment:

- how great were the concerns of maternity staff about fetal wellbeing in labour?

- do the cord gases suggest severe acidosis?

- was the baby floppy, extremely bradycardic and without any respiratory effort at birth?

- how long did the baby take to respond to resuscitation?

- were chest compressions used?

- was gasping seen at any stage?

- is the baby preterm, small for gestational age or growth restricted?

- how is the baby now? What is the tone, response, heart rate, breathing?

Observation is also warranted for babies who are at risk of infection, or from the side effects of maternal medication. Less commonly, babies with prenatally diagnosed disorders may need to be more closely monitored in the period after birth.

(d) Remaining with mother

If the decision is that the baby should remain with the mother, a clear plan of management should be documented and should include advice to feed early and specify the need to observe temperature, pulse and respirations on a regular basis. A structured early warning

system chart (such as that recently launched by the British Association of Perinatal Medicine called a 'Newborn Early Warning Trigger & Track" or 'NEWTT' score chart) [284] can be helpful in providing clear guidance on when to seek review and will help to avoid any deterioration being missed. [285, 286] The length of the observation period depends on the clinical status and can range from several minutes to a few hours as babies transition. In most cases, problems with transition resolve fairly quickly after birth, and the period of more intensive observation can be safely concluded without resorting to admission to the neonatal unit.

(e) Transfer to the neonatal unit

Continuing observation is necessary for any baby requiring resuscitation who then continues to have abnormal signs or symptoms, especially if there is a need for ongoing support.

When moving the baby for transfer, the baby should be kept warm, the airway controlled and any intravenous lines secured. Appropriate transport equipment should be used. If possible oxygen saturation should be monitored during transfer. The needs of the parents should be considered, ensuring that they are fully informed of events, the reasons for transfer and on-going care.

> **ENSURE THAT THE BABY IS WEARING THEIR IDENTITY BRACELETS BEFORE THEY LEAVE THE DELIVERY AREA**

In any situation, complete the notes as soon as possible. Record the baby's condition at birth, the resuscitation sequence and the baby's response to that resuscitation. Ensure that an explanation of the sequence of events is given to parents and document what they have been told.

Determining the root cause of the problem

(a) Acute hypoxia

The prognosis for the full term baby subjected to a sudden acute hypoxic insult (as a result, for example, of sudden immediately diagnosed cord prolapse or shoulder dystocia) can be very good, provided the episode does not last too long. Occasionally, however, even though the circulation is rapidly and effectively restored, cerebral function is very slow to recover.

The length of time it takes for reflex gasping activity to return gives some indication of the magnitude of the cerebral insult, but the length of time it takes for regular rhythmic (medullary) breathing to recover once the circulation is restored is a much more easily recorded event that gives a very good index of the severity of the cerebral insult.

Many of the babies who start to breathe again regularly within twenty minutes of the circulation being restored will recover completely but it is much rarer for a baby who is still only gasping after thirty minutes to recover. The majority die within days and almost all the documented survivors have severe spastic quadriplegia and profound learning difficulties from widespread generalised death of brain tissue. [250]

Many healthy survivors show cerebral irritability for a few days and some have fits, but few will show any other features and abnormal signs usually subside quickly.

The prognosis for a preterm baby less than 34 weeks gestation subjected to severe acute hypoxia is more unpredictable. There is a risk of secondary intraventricular haemorrhage or periventricular intracerebral haemorrhage and/or infarction after even a relatively brief severe hypoxic episode, especially in the crucial period immediately before and after birth.

Ultrasound scans give some indication of the position and size of the lesion but less indication of the amount of damage done. Many major lesions cause surprisingly few symptoms at the time, but can become apparent 7–10 days or more following the insult.

Babies with major lesions on cerebral ultrasound are at risk of severe developmental delay. However the correlation between the initial appearances and eventual outcome may not be sufficiently sensitive to be singularly predictive of poor outcome and thus may not be helpful in decisions regarding appropriate continuation of intensive care. Similarly, normal scans are not reassuring if the clinical picture suggests a poor prognosis.

(b) Chronic intra-uterine hypoxia

Chronic intra-uterine hypoxia, can cause aspiration of vernix or meconium deep into the lung, put the cardiac musculature under severe strain, promote hypertrophy of muscle within pulmonary arterioles, [156] or cause significant renal damage. It can cause serious cerebral ischaemia or haemorrhage, especially in the preterm baby. In the term baby, ischaemia can cause secondary cerebral oedema after a short, and deceptively encouraging, latent period. Normal labour and delivery is a significantly hypoxic experience for the fetus. Both the fetus and newborn baby withstand moderate chronic hypoxia (lack of oxygen) and asphyxia (lack of oxygen with a build-up of carbon dioxide) well.

Severe chronic intra-uterine hypoxia appears to be more damaging than acute severe hypoxia. The analogy is that sudden severe hypoxia stops the 'engine' abruptly whereas chronic fuel starvation, associated with severe chronic intra-uterine hypoxia, 'wrecks the machinery' before the 'engine' finally fails. This chronic intra-uterine hypoxia risks secondary cerebral oedema and apoptosis, and is associated with reperfusion injury. This may cause more damage than the original period of hypoxia itself. In addition, although the fetal heart (with a large reserve of glycogen) is remarkably resistant to acute hypoxic stress, chronic intra-uterine hypoxia may damage the myocardium resulting in low cardiac output. [287, 288] This has secondary consequences for other organs [13] particularly the kidney, which may develop 'pre-renal' failure due to poor perfusion, or acute tubular necrosis, if that hypoperfusion has been severe.

An electroencephalogram (EEG) can be helpful but requires expert interpretation to be useful. An amplitude-integrated EEG, or cerebral function monitor (CFM), may be easier to use and is more readily available in many neonatal units. Recent large doses of anticonvulsants will make interpretation even more difficult. Long-term prognosis depends largely on the depth of the post-hypoxic coma, the extent of any secondary cerebral oedema, and the severity and persistence of any seizure activity.

The extent of cerebral injury becomes more apparent following assessment over 36–48 h following an acute hypoxic insult. A mild short-lasting state of hyper-excitability usually carries a good prognosis even if there is seizure activity, but more severe symptoms can be associated with more severe developmental delay.

A quarter of babies with hypotonia and suppression of normal primitive reflex activity (Grade II encephalopathy in the classification of Sarnat and Sarnat summarised on p 80), suffer moderate developmental delay. The prognosis is worse if there are seizures. Most babies who are flaccid and stuporose (Grade III) will not survive, and if they do survive risk moderate to severe developmental delay. [289]

(c) Discriminating between primary and terminal apnoea

There is no instant way of determining if a baby is in primary apnoea and, therefore, merely needs a clear airway, or in terminal apnoea and needing active help. An Apgar score is frequently retrospective (and sometimes subjective) and indicates how unresponsive the baby is (which in turn may be due to shock, maternal sedation or simply immaturity rather than hypoxia). A cord pH only quantifies acidosis at that moment. Observation of the sequence of events during recovery will provide more information regarding cause of unresponsiveness. The brain's response during recovery is the only index of how far the process had progressed.

As oxygen returns to the brain the various control centres recover. As the baby responds it will exhibit changes in behaviour in reverse order to that shown as it deteriorated, which should help to determine how far the baby had deteriorated. Babies who have been in terminal apnoea do not cough or gasp until the circulation is restored and always exhibit a period of gasping before the onset of normal breathing movements. [1, 82]

(d) Umbilical cord blood gases

If there are concerns that the baby has been significantly compromised cord blood should be taken for measurement of pH, base deficit and lactate. Ideally, from an umbilical artery as well as from the umbilical vein (i.e. a 'paired' blood gas). [290-293] Both arterial and venous umbilical cord blood gas status is easily determined if two clamps are put on a 10 cm segment of the cord a minute after birth and the isolated portion put aside. Ideally these should be sampled and processed within 10 min. Blood pH estimation in samples from double-clamped vessels is reliable for up to 60 min but measurements of lactate are only reliable if analysed within 20 min. [290]

(e) Labelling the placenta for later examination

Detailed examination of the placenta, including a histological examination, may provide vital evidence regarding the reason why a baby required resuscitation at birth. The placenta should be labelled and histopathological examination requested. Placental pathological diagnoses can suggest aetiologies such as metabolic disorders, adverse growth events and infections as well as an alternative explanation for neonatal encephalopathy other than acute intrapartum hypoxia. [294]

(f) Kleihauer test

If a baby is born with significant anaemia, feto-maternal haemorrhage should be considered as a differential diagnosis. It is important to request that a sample of blood is taken from the mother and a Kleihauer test requested (which tests for evidence of feto-maternal bleeding). The Keihauer (sometimes called Kleihauer-Betke) test detects fetal cells, which contain HbF, in the maternal blood. [295]

(g) Sepsis

Sepsis should **always** be considered as a possible underlying cause for, and may be the primary reason for, fetal distress. If this is a possibility, cultures should be taken and treatment commenced within 1 h of consideration of this diagnosis. [296] The placenta should be sent for later histological examination as above.

Later post-resuscitation care

A number of complications may occur after an anoxic insult. Though they may occur after a profound but acute insult, they are much more common after a less profound but prolonged insult.

(a) Respiratory depression

Some babies may need continuing ventilation following a hypoxic insult. Blood gases will need to be monitored and transfer to an intensive care unit will need to be arranged.

- **Blood gas monitoring**: Beware over-ventilation. Respiratory acidosis can be treated by increasing ventilatory support. However, it is easy to over ventilate a baby with normal lungs, and important to avoid hypocarbia and hyperoxaemia. Reducing the $PaCO_2$ below 4 kPa reduces cerebral perfusion and is strongly associated with neurological damage. [281, 297] There is also evidence that hyperoxaemia is also associated with increased damage, especially if combined with hypocarbia. [298]

- **Oxygen saturation monitoring:** Continuous monitoring of oxygenation is important. Persistent pulmonary hypertension of the newborn (PPHN), with blood by-passing the lung through the foramen ovale and/or ductus arteriosus, can rapidly become a serious problem if not detected and treated promptly. Monitoring pre- and post-ductal oxygen saturations is very useful in the initial assessment of PPHN with a difference of 5% or more being significant. Appropriate ventilation and oxygenation may reduce the likelihood of this occurring. Early accurate diagnosis and treatment of this rare problem is likely to require echocardiographic investigation.

(b) Cardiac function monitoring

A transient post-hypoxic cardiomyopathy is common and blood pressure monitoring is important. If myocardial function is compromised, treating any hypotension with one of more boluses of fluid may be detrimental. Similarly premature babies may have impaired cardiac function due to the increased after-load on the heart which early birth entails. [299] Echocardiographic assessment of cardiac function (functional echocardiography), if available, should be used to guide appropriate use of inotropic support.

(c) Metabolic acidosis

Virtually all babies who have been in terminal apnoea will have a degree of metabolic acidosis. Once the circulation is restored and respiration (or at least gaseous exchange) is established, this will be corrected over a period of several hours by the baby's lungs and kidneys. Though bicarbonate is very occasionally used during resuscitation if there is no cardiac output despite chest compressions, it is rarely required following successful resuscitation (Chapter 7). Slow partial correction of a metabolic acidosis may occasionally be useful in certain circumstances, for example, in very immature babies, because a pH below 7.2 inhibits surfactant production. Even in these situations there is no need for rapid correction, and calculated correction could be given over 6–12 h. Correction may also be appropriate as part of the treatment strategy if the baby is developing signs of persistent pulmonary hypertension with right-to-left shunting. In general, however, it is best to allow the baby to correct this by itself.

(d) Renal function monitoring

Renal function is often impaired following significant intrapartum hypoxia. Total fluid intake should be restricted to a minimum (40–60 mL kg^{-1} per day) until renal function recovers. Antibiotic dosing frequency should also be adjusted if renal function is reduced.

- **Urine output:** Monitor urine output closely. Urine may be present in the bladder at the time of the insult and so initial urine output may be normal. Urine should be examined for blood, protein, pH and cellular debris.

- **Daily weighing of baby** is useful in monitoring fluid balance.

- **Sodium:** Monitor urinary and sodium closely for hyponatraemia. Assess whether it is due to (a) oliguria and water retention, (b) cellular damage causing sodium redistribution within the body, or (c) renal loss of sodium, before attempting treatment. Measuring sodium and creatinine levels in both plasma and urine will allow calculation fractional sodium excretion.

- **Glucose:** Blood glucose levels may be either too low or too high. Continuous glucose infusion will be required. Usually 10% glucose is used, however, it may if be necessary to use a more concentrated solution to maintain blood glucose when low fluid volumes are being infused.

(e) Medications

The combination of impaired renal and hepatic function can adversely impact on the metabolism of many drugs used in the baby recovering from a hypoxic insult. In addition, therapeutic hypothermia (see below) may further slow the metabolism of many of the drugs that are metabolised by liver enzymes and dose adjustments may be needed both during the hypothermia and re-warming periods. [300]

Therapeutic hypothermia

Evidence from animal studies has shown that cooling the brain reduces the secondary damage that occurs in the hours after a hypoxic insult and this approach has now gained widespread acceptance as a treatment for infants with moderately severe hypoxic ischaemic encephalopathy (HIE). Whilst the emphasis is on maintaining normothermia **during** resuscitation, there is some evidence that the earlier therapeutic hypothermia is considered and started the better the outcome.

Hyperthermia (defined in this instance as a temperature ≥38.0°C), particularly when induced by external heating, is to be avoided at all costs in babies who have suffered perinatal brain injury. Following resuscitation, the overhead heater on the resuscitaire should be switched off if therapeutic hypothermia is considered.

(a) When to consider therapeutic hypothermia

Perinatal hypoxia severe enough to cause HIE is estimated to occur in approximately 1–6 per 1000 births. [301, 302] It creates a major burden for the individual, the family and for society. [303] Following the results of three randomised controlled trials, including the UK total body cooling (TOBY) trial [89], it was confirmed that 72 h of cooling to a core temperature of 33–34 °C started within six hours of birth reduces death and disability at 18 months of age. Targeted therapeutic hypothermia

improves a range of neurodevelopmental outcomes in survivors. [89-91] Following a meta-analysis of these data [92] the treatment was recommended by the National Institute for Health and Care Excellence (NICE) as it is cost-effective in the context of the National Health Service (NICE IPG374) [304] and is supported by the British Association of Perinatal Medicine (BAPM). [305]

(b) When to initiate therapeutic hypothermia

In the UK the criteria for deciding which babies to treat with therapeutic hypothermia have largely been adopted, with minor local variations, from those used in the TOBY trial. [89] These state that infants in the following categories may be considered for treatment:

- ≥36 weeks completed gestation

- require resuscitation at birth

- develop seizures or moderate or severe encephalopathy after resuscitation.

Babies in the above groups are then assessed against additional criteria (criteria A and B):

Criteria A

Infants who fall into the above groups and who are admitted to the neonatal unit meet criteria A if they have **at least one** of the following:

- Apgar score of ≤5 at 10 min after birth

- Continued need for resuscitation, including endotracheal or mask ventilation, at 10 min after birth

- Acidosis within 60 min of birth (defined as any occurrence of umbilical cord, arterial or capillary pH <7.00)

- Base Deficit ≥ 16 mmol L^{-1} in umbilical cord or any blood sample (arterial, venous or capillary) within 60 min of birth

Infants that meet criteria A are then assessed to see whether they meet the neurological abnormality entry criteria (criteria B):

Criteria B

- Seizures, or

- Moderate to severe encephalopathy, consisting of:

  - altered state of consciousness (reduced response to stimulation or absent response to stimulation), and,

  - abnormal tone (focal or general hypotonia, or flaccid), and,

  - abnormal primitive reflexes (weak or absent suck or Moro response)

Treatment with therapeutic hypothermia should be considered in infants who have met both criteria A and B.

When cooling is initiated (either active or passive), this should be done in accordance with the network guidelines and local care pathways and after discussion with their designated network neonatal intensive care unit (NICU). Some neonatal networks have agreed extended inclusion and exclusion criteria.

The BAPM position statement [305] includes a general point regarding the use of therapeutic hypothermia in infants who did not fit the clinical trial criteria:

'No data currently supports the use of cooling for neuroprotection in infants of lower gestational age or for other conditions such as sudden postnatal collapse or seizures thought to be due to acute cerebral infarction. Clinicians who choose to cool in these situations should be aware of the weak evidence basis for treatment in these circumstances and parents should be informed of this before treatment is started.'

Amplitude integrated EEG or cerebral function monitoring, is helpful for obtaining evidence of cerebral depression and active therapeutic hypothermia should not be undertaken in a centre that cannot monitor cerebral activity. Anticonvulsants should be administered if there is seizure activity.

(c) Passive cooling

Once a decision has been made to offer cooling, if equipment for active cooling is not available, passive cooling can be started while arrangements are made to transfer the baby to a cooling centre. Passive cooling requires monitoring of rectal temperature but its use helps to avoid delays in starting treatment that would otherwise occur. [306]

Longer term prognosis

(a) Apgar Score of 0 for ≥ 10 min

Despite the short-comings of the Apgar score (Appendix 1), a score of 0 at 10 min is a strong predictor of mortality and morbidity in both late preterm and term infants. If the heart rate remains undetectable after 10 min of resuscitation, it may be reasonable to consider stopping resuscitation; however the decision to continue or discontinue should be individualised taking into account whether the resuscitation was considered to be optimal, availability of advanced neonatal care (e.g. the availability of therapeutic hypothermia), specific circumstances prior to delivery (e.g., known timing of the insult) and wishes expressed by the family.

(b) Predicting death or disability of newborn infants >34 weeks based on Apgar and/or absence of breathing

Absence of spontaneous breathing or an Apgar score of 1 to 3 at 20 min of age in babies born at >34 weeks

gestation but with a detectable heart rate are strong predictors of mortality or significant morbidity. In settings where resources are limited it is suggested that it may be reasonable to stop assisted ventilation. In areas where neonatal intensive care, including the use of ventilation and therapeutic hypothermia, is available the decision to stop resuscitation may be much less clear and local senior advice should be sought. The specific circumstances prior to delivery (e.g. known timing of the insult), and wishes expressed by the family should be taken into account when making this decision.

The initial state of the baby is less important than the speed with which they respond to resuscitation once it is started. The speed with which the neurological signs improve is more significant than the speed with which respiration and the circulation recover. Seizures are poor prognostic features and babies requiring ventilatory support for respiratory depression have an extremely bad prognosis. It is justifiable to offer continuing support where aspiration, pneumonia or seizures (and/or treatment thereof) jeopardise respiratory exchange.

Therapeutic hypothermia has significantly altered the prognosis for babies with moderate, though not severe, encephalopathy. If started within six hours of birth, it reduces death and disability at 18 months of age and improves a range of neurodevelopmental outcomes in survivors. Other therapeutic strategies involving erythropoietin, magnesium sulfate, melatonin, topiramate and xenon ventilation remain under investigation. [307]

Communication and record keeping

(a) In an emergency, structured communication helps

Communication problems are a factor in up to 80% of adverse incidents or near miss reports in hospitals. Failure of communication is also evident when a newborn emergency occurs and a doctor, nurse or midwife summons senior help. The caller often fails to communicate the seriousness of the situation or conveys the information in a way that fails to ensure that the recipient appreciates the urgency of the situation. A well-structured process that is simple, reliable and dependable will enable the caller to convey the important facts, the degree of urgency and allow the recipient to plan ahead.

Use of the acronym, SBAR (Situation-Background-Assessment-Recommendation) is helpful in planning effective, timely communication between individuals from different clinical backgrounds and hierarchies. It is recommended that this format is used in all cases.

Using imprecise communication during the resuscitation introduces the opportunity for misunderstanding and misinterpretation among team members, and increases the chances for errors to occur. For example, *"Someone get me some adrenaline"* can result in the incorrect dose being given or the drug being given by the incorrect route. It is far better to state " *Staff nurse Smith, I would like you to draw up adrenaline, 1:10 000 concentration, 0.3 mL for the umbilical venous catheter.*" This clarifies for whom the order is intended, as well as the desired medication, dose, concentration, and route of administration. This communication should be completed by the person fulfilling the order: "*Here is the adrenaline, 1:10 000 concentration, 0.3 mL for the umbilical venous catheter*", thus closing the loop of communication. [308]

(b) Written records

Accurate and comprehensive records are crucial, particularly in resuscitation at birth where records may be carefully scrutinised years later. Ideally, case notes should be prepared prior to the birth to allow for information to be collated in advance. If case notes are not available then the scraps of paper used to note down information during resuscitation may be attached to the case notes as they constitute a contemporaneous record of what took place. [309] Overall the record should '*be factual and not include unnecessary abbreviations, jargon, meaningless phrases or irrelevant speculation.*' [310]

- **Facts not opinions:** Accurate written record should document all that happened as soon as possible after an event. Words used in such a record should be carefully considered and it should be remembered that these could be used in a court of law. The records may assume considerable medico-legal importance in later years. Fact must be distinguished from opinion, and the appropriateness of any adjective should be carefully considered. What was seen and done should be recorded and there must be no assumptions made as to causation.

  Facts relating to the birth (e.g. fetal bradycardia, non-reassuring cardiotocograph (CTG) trace, low scalp pH) should be noted. The time of every event should be noted as accurately as possible. Words such as '*asphyxia*' and '*fetal distress*' should not be used as they are impossible to define in this context. [311] The term '*flat baby*' is particularly unhelpful whether spoken or written. Any reference to the obstetric handling of the case should be purely factual.

- **What to record:** After any resuscitation the following information should be recorded:

  - when you were called, by whom, and why
  - the time you arrived, who else was there, and the condition of the baby on your arrival
  - what you did, when you did it, and the timing and details of any response from the baby. Recording these in sequence is helpful
  - whether the baby was floppy and whether they were conscious at birth
  - the baby's heart rate at birth and when it first became fast (i.e. exceeded 100 min[-1])
  - the time when you were first certain that the lungs had been successfully inflated

  - whether gasping respiration preceded the onset of rhythmical breathing, when gasping started and how long it lasted
  - when the baby started to breathe evenly, regularly and effectively 30–60 min[-1] (even if gasping is still occurring intermittently)
  - if you have used a saturation monitor it is helpful to note the initial reading of both the heart rate and saturations and how these changed with you actions.
  - the date and time of writing your entry followed by your name, your role and grade, your signature and your professional registration number.

(c) Communication with other professionals

Where a problem has been suspected antenatally or during labour, it should be communicated to the neonatal staff so that an appropriate plan of action can be drawn up (Appendix 4).

If the problem is diagnosed in the postnatal period then the general practitioner, community midwife, health visitor and other members of the primary health care team should be informed. The obstetrician and midwife responsible for the mother's care should also be informed. A telephone call may be appropriate to ensure a speedy exchange of information, rather than waiting for formally produced letters and memos. This can be followed up with a letter or note confirming the information. Conversations should be documented carefully and should include details of the persons concerned, the content of the exchange and the date and time.

(d) Communication with parents

It is important to remember that the parents are the people to whom all information about their child should be primarily directed. Ideally the information should be shared with both parents together and only with their explicit permission should information be given to others. Very occasionally circumstances may arise where information has to be shared with other family members first but this will be a very rare event.

The birth of a child is an exceptionally important event for parents and they will be extremely anxious if their baby receives any resuscitation at birth. Always speak to the parents as soon as possible; before birth if circumstances allow and it is thought that resuscitation is likely to be needed. They will assume the worst even if their baby was only on the resuscitaire for a few minutes. Parents often fear that any baby receiving resuscitation is likely to be 'brain-damaged'. Let them see, touch and hold their baby even if the baby is going to the neonatal unit. However, don't let the baby get cold or hypoxic in the process.

Information given to parents or other family members about the baby and any possible outcomes should be objective and should avoid prejudging care. In particular, the person responsible for resuscitation is not usually in a position to make an informed comment on the management of the pregnancy or labour and delivery. This should be left for midwifery and obstetric staff to deal with. Any discussions with parents should be documented.

Stressful situations can inhibit the retention of information and the use of jargon may further complicate the situation. Check the parents' understanding of the information you have given them by asking them to explain what they think you mean. It is the job of professionals to explain effectively.

(e) Language or other communication barriers

Some parents may have difficulties with communication because of disability or language problems. In these situations interpreters may have to be used. Using other family members to translate important information is generally bad practice as they may not understand the information they are being asked to give, they may translate the information inaccurately and you risk breaching patient confidentiality. Any information communicated to the parents should be clearly documented and this record should include a note of the parents' reaction to the information and any questions that they ask.

When a decision is made not to resuscitate a baby, the parents should be closely involved and in agreement with the decision. The reasons for the decision should be documented, along with a record of the discussion with the parents and their reaction.

Summary learning

- A baby who has been resuscitated is at risk of further deterioration and post resuscitation plans should consider this.

- Placental pathology and blood tests from mother may help in elucidating the underlying cause of the baby's problems.

- If sepsis is considered, antibiotics should be administered within one hour.

- If a baby is not admitted to a neonatal unit there should be a clear plan for further observation and review.

- A baby admitted to the neonatal unit post resuscitation should have vital signs and biochemistry monitored with appropriate interventions to maintain stability.

- Therapeutic hypothermia (cooling) should be considered in babies who are in very poor condition at birth and who demonstrate signs of hypoxic ischaemic encephalopathy.

- Parents and other professionals should be communicated with clearly and appropriately. Detailed notes of what is said to the family and when must be clearly documented in the medical records.

- Medical records should be clear, detailed, factual, legible, timed, dated and signed.

My key take-home messages from this chapter

Babies who do not respond

Contents

- **The most common reasons for failure to respond to resuscitative efforts and ways to address these**
- **When to consider ceasing resuscitative efforts and the situations in which it might be decided not to start**
- **The legal definitions of live birth and stillbirth after resuscitation and at low gestations.**

Learning outcomes

To enable you to:

- **Discuss the possible reasons why a baby might not respond to the standard approach**
- **Describe the techniques that might be used to treat these unusual cases**
- **Understand when it may be appropriate to stop resuscitation or inappropriate to begin**

Considerations when a baby's heart rate doesn't respond after the standard approach

The commonest reason for a baby's heart rate failing to improve is inadequate management of airway and breathing. In this situation make sure to check:

- Is the baby's head in the neutral position?
- Do you need a second person's help with the airway?
- Do you need jaw thrust?
- Are you using a 2–3 s inflation time?

If all of these are being achieved, consider:

- Is there an obstruction in the airway? (laryngoscope and suction)
- Is an airway needed (either oropharyngeal or laryngeal mask airway)?

Material blocking the trachea

Lumps of vernix, blood clot, thick mucus or particulate meconium, if large enough, can obstruct the trachea if inhaled. Any such inhalation will almost always have occurred as the result of gasping *in utero*. If, using the standard approach outlined previously, you cannot aerate the lungs despite using a well-fitting mask, consider the possibility of impacted debris in the trachea. Tracheal intubation for suctioning should be considered where there is no increase in heart rate and no chest movement with mask ventilation. [17, 18] If you are not trained to intubate, look into the mouth with a laryngoscope and ensure that the oropharynx is clear. At this point, consider use of either higher inflation pressures or longer inflation times aiming to get some air into the airway pending the arrival of someone who can intubate.

NLS

Pneumothorax

If care is taken to limit the inflation pressure used then pneumothorax is a rare cause of problems at birth. It is not always necessary to drain a pneumothorax in the delivery room and directly aspirating the chest with a syringe and butterfly needle on the faint suspicion of a pneumothorax may well produce one. There may be antenatal information available to suggest that a pneumothorax is more likely to occur during the course of resuscitation (e.g. if the baby is known to have pulmonary hypoplasia on antenatal scans).

In the very rare situation of a tension pneumothorax – suggested by a cyanosed baby, with bradycardia, who does not respond to ventilation and who has reduced breath sounds on one side – more urgent drainage may be needed using needle thoracocentesis (Appendix 2).

If possible it is best to transfer the baby to the neonatal unit and confirm the diagnosis by X-ray or by examination with a 'cold-light' before treatment.

Stiff lungs

In some cases the lungs may be unusually stiff (non-compliant). This might occur in situations where severe oligohydramnios or anhydramnios has led to pulmonary hypoplasia. In these cases, despite the manoeuvres discussed above it may not be possible to adequately inflate the lungs and oxygenate the baby. If the clinical situation suggests that stiff lungs may be a contributory factor, and you are confident that the airway is open, it may also be worth considering increasing the peak inflation pressure.

This initial period of increased pressure may be sufficient to exceed the higher critical opening pressure of the stiffer lung and enable lung inflation to occur. Once inflated, the pressures required to continue with ventilatory support may be lower. If suitable equipment is available, you should measure the tidal volumes to guide you to the pressures required and be prepared to reduce the pressures as soon as possible. There is an increased risk of air leak/pneumothorax with such stiffer lungs, especially with higher pressures.

The baby who is pale, shocked, dyspnoeic or hypovolaemic

If chest wall movement has been confirmed and the heart rate does not respond, chest compressions can be commenced, as outlined previously. While most resuscitation situations will only require one or two cycles of chest compressions to move oxygenated blood back to the heart to improve heart rate, some infants will have a persistent bradycardia despite subsequent intravenous drug administration. In this situation, hypovolaemia should be suspected. In some situations, the obstetric team may be able to provide information before or during delivery that raises the index of suspicion of hypovolaemia earlier in resuscitation.

Hypovolaemic shock at delivery is rare and results from acute, peripartum blood loss. It can occur with placental abruption, or after acute feto-maternal bleeding. Cutting through an anterior placenta during caesarean section can cause fetal blood loss. A ruptured placental vessel (vasa praevia) can easily be missed, as can blood loss into the baby's own abdominal cavity from trauma to the spleen or liver. Partial umbilical cord occlusion may obstruct blood flow through the umbilical vein but not the umbilical arteries (where the blood is at higher pressure) resulting in blood reaching the placenta but failing to return to the baby. A similar problem may follow shoulder dystocia, particularly if the cord is cut before the baby is extracted.

Treatment of hypovolaemia involves passing an umbilical venous catheter (if not already done). A sample of blood for Hb (baseline), cross-matching and 1 spot on the newborn blood spot ("Guthrie") card, for pre-transfusion haemoglobinopathy screening, should be taken if possible. Volume replacement can initially be provided with 10 mL kg^{-1} of 0.9% sodium chloride or colloid solution (10 mL kg^{-1} is equivalent to giving a 70 kg adult a bolus of 700 mL of IV fluid). Later 20–40 mL kg^{-1} of blood may be required. Unmatched group O Rhesus (D) negative blood is entirely appropriate, and it should be easily available in an emergency, from a locally agreed central location (e.g. main theatre or the emergency department). In the longer term the need for further blood can be assessed by watching for a progressive fall in haematocrit and the umbilical venous catheter (if close to the right atrium) is ideal for measuring central venous pressure.

The baby who remains blue

If the baby remains blue but has an acceptable heart rate, check for possible airway problems listed above. Keep ventilating and call for help. Use a pulse oximeter to check the pre-ductal oxygen saturation if not already applied. Other causes of continued cyanosis in a normal looking term baby are very rare. They include undiagnosed diaphragmatic hernia and intrapartum pneumonia. It is rare for congenital cyanotic heart disease to be obvious this early though some cyanosis is present from birth. Duskiness can be the first sign of persistent pulmonary hypertension, which can easily spiral rapidly out of control if not recognised and treated quickly. You should be able to achieve 100% saturation in 100% oxygen if there is no right-to-left shunt.

> **CONTINUED CYANOSIS AND LOW OXYGEN SATURATIONS REQUIRE IMMEDIATE INVESTIGATION AND SENIOR HELP**

Narcotics and naloxone

Babies affected by opiates given to the mother usually cry at birth, but may become apnoeic when wrapped up warm and comfortable a few minutes later. [312] The baby most at risk is one whose mother has had repeated doses of opiates less than three hours apart (the adult half-life), who has had intravenous (IV) rather than intramuscular (IM) doses, or who has received the drug less than 2–3 h before delivery. If a baby is apnoeic secondary to maternal opiates the priority is for lung aeration and subsequent ventilation. Only when the airway is secure, lung aeration has been achieved, the baby is ventilated or breathing and heart rate is normal, should naloxone treatment be considered. Naloxone is **not** an emergency drug and is not given during resuscitation but rather once the baby is stable from a cardiovascular perspective but remains apnoeic due to maternal opiate administration.

Babies who are apnoeic secondary to maternal opiates should, once their airway (A), breathing (B) and circulation (C) have been addressed, be given 200 micrograms of intramuscular (IM) naloxone (0.5 mL of the standard 400 microgram/mL ampoule or Minijet®). Smaller doses (such as that obtainable from 2 mL vials of 20 microgram/mL ampoules) will also reverse the sedation but the effect of this will only last a short time; approximately 20 min if given intravenously and a few hours if given intramuscularly. This is insufficient to counter the effect of pethidine, for example, which can last for more than 24 h in the exposed newborn infant. Narcotics accumulate progressively in the unborn baby after administration to the mother.

Hydrops fetalis

Hydrops fetalis is a condition in the fetus characterised by an accumulation of fluid, or oedema, in at least two fetal compartments (e.g. the pleural, pericardial or peritoneal cavities and/or the skin). It is a condition that brings particular challenges to the delivery room. It is usually diagnosed by antenatal ultrasound, although it may rarely be an unexpected finding at delivery in which case it should prompt an immediate call for senior assistance. Being aware of the diagnosis can allow the neonatal team useful opportunity to prepare a strategy for resuscitating the baby with hydrops in advance of delivery. The baby will be pale and bloated with generalised oedema, ascites and occasionally pleural effusions. It may be necessary to drain the abdominal ascites (from the left iliac fossa, to avoid damage to an enlarged liver or spleen) and apply an airway pressure of more than 30 cm water in order to achieve better diaphragmatic movement and lung aeration. If this does not work, drainage of pleural effusions should then be considered to optimise lung aeration. Pleural effusions only occasionally interfere with lung aeration.

Ascitic or pleural fluid is best drained with a relatively wide bore needle or cannula (e.g. 20 gauge). In the very rare event that volume expansion is needed following drainage of either ascitic or pleural fluid, a crystalloid is preferred. Albumin or blood is relatively contraindicated because it can raise the intravascular osmolality significantly resulting in rapid influx of tissue fluid and added myocardial strain. For the same reason it may be important to consider leaving a modest volume deficit after exchange transfusion.

When should you stop?

The neonatal group within the International Liaison Committee on Resuscitation (ILCOR), in its most recent review of the published evidence, addressed this question. [17] The best available data is of moderate quality with small numbers of infants. Whilst there is evidence of better outcomes with the use of therapeutic hypothermia; infants who are ≥36 weeks at birth with an Apgar score of 0 at 10 min still, as a group, have a poor prognosis. Studies showed that of the ~50% who survive delivery room resuscitation, 76% either died before the age of 22 months old or had moderate to severe neurodevelopmental impairment. [313-315] Thus around a quarter of these infants survived without moderate to severe neurological sequelae however there is a great deal of 'selection bias' in that treatment is only offered to those babies who are alive after resuscitation.

The current NLS recommendation is that if the heart rate is not detectable at birth and remains undetectable for 10 min (equivalent to an Apgar score of zero at 10 min) despite resuscitation, it may be appropriate to **consider** stopping resuscitation as this situation is highly predictive of death or severe morbidity for the baby. However, the decision to continue or withhold resuscitative efforts should be individualised at the time of resuscitation and involve senior advice. The availability of on-going advanced neonatal intensive care (including therapeutic hypothermia), specific circumstances prior to delivery (e.g. known timing of the insult), and wishes expressed by the family should be taken into account when making this decision.

Whether, or when, to stop resuscitation in a baby whose heart rate is present but remains below 60 min⁻¹ after 10 min is much less clear and local senior advice should be sought. Absence of spontaneous breathing or an Apgar score one to three at 20 min of age, in babies >34 weeks gestation but with a detectable heart rate, are strong predictors of mortality or significant morbidity. [17, 18]

There are also situations where the more pertinent question is 'should resuscitation even be attempted?' ILCOR has tried to address this question also. Clearly there are groups of babies defined by gestation, birth weight or the presence of specific congenital anomalies, that are associated with almost certain death or else rare survival but with very high morbidity and in these cases it is reasonable not to attempt resuscitation. However, what is perhaps more important is for local obstetric and neonatal teams to have developed a consistent approach to this problem in the light of local conditions and which takes into account the views of the parents. [316, 317]

Extreme prematurity

It is rare for a baby significantly less than 500 grams at birth to survive, but many show signs of life after birth. [318-320] Such signs may persist for several hours in some extremely immature infants. [321] It is dishonest and hurtful to brush aside such signs of life and classify the baby as stillborn, especially when the family has witnessed these signs.

Most parents value having the opportunity to see and hold their dead or dying baby. Parents can readily understand that their baby is in the process of dying and can be grateful for the chance to share in this if reassured that the laboured gasps are not a sign of conscious pain or distress. They will want to be confident that the baby was assessed and that any chance of survival was not dismissed out of hand. It can be a comfort to stress that parent's love, care, comfort and warmth were the most important contributions to their baby's short life.

To handle this situation with sensitivity and skill calls for experience. Therefore, junior members of staff should not be left to face such situations without support. A framework for clinical practice endorsed by the British Association of Perinatal Medicine (BAPM) has been published. [317]

Each department should agree a guideline for planning and managing births at extremely low gestational ages. You should familiarise yourself with your local guidelines but if you are in doubt about whether to intervene you should start resuscitation and get a senior colleague to come and assist you immediately. [322]

Definitions of live birth and stillbirth

It is important for families that when a baby dies, the classification of its death is made correctly. Incorrect classification, or disagreement (such as that between obstetricians and paediatricians about the presence or absence of signs of life) can cause distress and suffering for newly bereaved parents.

UK: The legal definition of a live birth in the UK is *"a child born alive"*. Note that no gestational age is mentioned in this definition.

The legal definition of a stillbirth is a little more helpful and is:

"A child which has issued forth from its mother after the 24th week of pregnancy and which did not at any time after being completely expelled from its mother breathe or show any other signs of life"

Note that in the UK, babies born dead before 24 completed weeks of gestation are not registered as stillbirths but babies who are born alive at any gestation should be registered as live births.

World Health Organisation: The World Health Organisation (WHO) definitions are a bit more informative. The WHO definition of a live birth is:

"the complete expulsion or extraction from its mother of a product of conception, irrespective of the duration of the pregnancy, which, after such separation, breathes or shows any other evidence of life, such as beating of the heart, pulsation of the umbilical cord, or definite movement of voluntary muscles, whether or not the umbilical cord has been cut or the placenta is attached; each product of such a birth is considered liveborn. Twins both born alive count as two live births but a child who dies from asphyxia caused by shoulder dystocia after delivery of the head but before delivery of the body is not a live birth."

The WHO does not use the term stillbirth but refers to fetal death. A fetal death is defined as:

"death prior to complete expulsion or extraction from its mother of a product of conception, irrespective of

the duration of pregnancy; the death is indicated by the fact that after such separation the fetus does not breathe or show any other evidence of life, such as beating of the heart, pulsation of the umbilical cord, or definite movement of voluntary muscles."

Summary learning

When babies fail to respond to the standard approach:

- **Call for senior help.**

- **Ensure that you are using all the skills you have learnt to keep the chest moving.**

- **Consider tracheal obstruction or pneumothorax if there is inadequate chest movement despite executing the standard approach properly.**

- **If all the above fail consider higher inflation pressures and/or longer inflation times.**

Then:

- **If bradycardia persists in the presence of adequate ventilation as judged by good chest movement, then start chest compressions.**

- **If the baby remains bradycardic administer adrenaline, bicarbonate and glucose via UVC.**

- **With persistent bradycardia or where there is known perinatal blood loss, consider immediate administration of volume or blood.**

- **Consider stopping resuscitation if the heart rate is still undetected after 10 min but ensure that you have called for senior help as this should not be a junior decision.**

My key take-home messages from this chapter

64

Non-technical skills

Contents

- **Communication**
- **Systems**
- **Processes**
- **Non-technical skills and decision making**

Learning outcomes

To enable you to:
- **Gain insight into the way individuals and teams work together during resuscitation situations**
- **Improve team communication**
- **Improve the management of resuscitation of the newborn through knowledge of individual and team dynamics**
- **Reflect upon personal attributes which may be relevant in any resuscitation situation**

Introduction

Resuscitation of a newborn baby can be a very stressful situation for anyone, especially if it is unexpected or prolonged. This can be exacerbated if those involved are inexperienced or unfamiliar with the staff, environment, procedures and processes necessary to effectively deal with matters.

In this chapter we shall discuss key elements which may be critical in the timely management of a potentially difficult situation. The likelihood of a successful outcome is improved if thought has been given beforehand to these issues, which are important not just in newborn resuscitation, but in any process.

Although effective teamwork is essential in prolonged or complicated resuscitations, for the vast majority of deliveries where any resuscitation is required there is no need for a 'team' as such; a single resuscitator providing good basic life support will resuscitate most babies before the rest of the team arrives.

Communication

We have already discussed in Chapter 5 how important structured communication is in resuscitation situations. The use of tools, such as SBAR [323, 324], facilitate clear communication between staff at all levels.

Language

There is a natural tendency to use jargon during professional dialogue. Whilst in many cases this is helpful in rapidly communicating complex issues, it is important to ensure that what has been said is understood. Do not assume everyone interprets things the same way. [308]

Effective resource management

Knowledge of the systems in place and how they work in advance of a resuscitation situation makes it much more likely to be managed properly. [325] Different units will have different ways of preparing for these situations; for example, identifying high risk births requiring medical attendance, using a standard protocol for summoning the correct emergency team, advertising fixed locations for crash trolleys, standardising the equipment stored on the resuscitaire and the layout of the delivery room or theatre. Being familiar with these and many other factors help ensure the smooth running of a situation.

> **PLANNING**
> **PREVENTS**
> **PROBLEMS**

Lack of knowledge, or application of systems in place, make it much more likely that problems will arise. Individually these might be an inconvenience, but the risk is that these 'inconveniences' combine to create a life-threatening crisis. [145-147, 325]

An example of the cumulative errors leading to a serious untoward event might be:

- An initial failure to recognise a high-risk pregnancy leading to the delivery of a baby requiring support without the medical team being present.

- The attendance of the medical team being delayed by a failure to invoke the correct emergency call.

- The medical team composed of junior doctors who have just rotated to that hospital and are unfamiliar with the hospital layout, and they are unsure exactly where the problem is because they have not been told which room when they were called.

- On arrival they find the equipment in the room has not been checked following a previous delivery and there is a delay in the arrival of the emergency trolley because an inexperienced member of staff does not know where to find it.

Thus a combination of events leads to potentially significant delays in managing the situation.

Process & procedures

The NLS algorithm is a good example of a process which ensures that all involved are aware of the sequence of events. They can anticipate needs, recognise omissions and be in a position to support. Knowledge of the sequence is vital, but equally important are practical skills. It is important not just enough to know when to undertake a manoeuvre but also to be able to do it competently.

Thus within the NLS it is expected that following assessment the airway is opened and if necessary inflation

breaths provided. It does not help if the airway opening manoeuvre is flawed, and inflation breaths poorly administered.

Non-technical skills & team working:

Individual factors and the dynamic of the team can significantly affect the outcome of resuscitation. [326] These non-technical attributes have been termed 'human factors' and include:

- Situational awareness

- Decision making

- Team working & leadership

- Task management

- Communication.

Situational awareness

Situational awareness describes the ability of an individual to retain a global overview of the situation. In newborn resuscitation those dealing with the baby are frequently managing the airway and may focus solely on this potentially to the exclusion of other important factors – so called 'fixation'. [145-147] In complex situations and where a team is available, it can be helpful to step back and delegate tasks in order to be able to consider the bigger picture. In doing so it is possible to co-ordinate more effectively, monitor progress and identify any issues which may not have been dealt with.

Whilst there is some evidence that situational awareness tends to correlate with expertise, this does not mean that the individual detects all important events. In one simple experiment, volunteers who were adult resuscitators were shown videos of a simulated cardiac arrest that included a series of change-events designed to elicit perceptual errors; approximately 80% of inexperienced and 60% of experienced resuscitators missed the fact that the patient's oxygen supply had become disconnected. [327]

Decision making

It is important that clear decisions are made, communicated and carried out in a timely manner, particularly in complex or prolonged resuscitations. The team leader should be a good communicator, be a good listener and be decisive. The team leader should also be able to manage conflict which involves any team member proposing or suggesting something different to that already communicated. Whilst such conflict may be helpful to raise issues, it can also raise tension and cause delay in decision making and damage the focus of the team or the team leader. Three levels of conflict have been described: [328]

(1) Discussion

Where a team member may communicate *awareness* of a procedure, an item of kit, a protocol or an available expert and this may result in *discussion*. Discussion can be helpful in that it permits examination of a problem and should be encouraged irrespective of role, seniority or experience. The team leader should then *acknowledge* the information, then assess it and *maybe* use it to accomplish the treatment goal.

(2) Disagreement

There may be *disagreement* over management. In this case the team leader should *acknowledge* the difference in opinion but must then be *decisive* after quickly exploring the alternative so as to minimise any delays.

(3) Dispute

Dispute is perhaps the most difficult situation in an already stressful situation. Again the team leader should *acknowledge* the difference of opinion, but then they need to *assert* their view and take action. If a team has a common goal (i.e. resuscitation of the baby) then conflict can usually be overcome by stressing the commitment to the common goal.

Most often it is enough to stress the extreme urgency of the situation and the need to work as a team where the performance of every team member contributes to the overall success of the resuscitation. It may be helpful to state that the dispute (or the attitude of the disputing person) is not helping. In an extreme situation where the dispute threatens to impede the process the team leader may ask someone to 'step out'.

Team working & leadership

Teams need to be organised with a clear leader. It can sometimes be helpful for the accepted team leader to become less practically involved with the resuscitation and more concerned with an oversight of the situation. The role of team leader is dynamic and depends on the skill mix and number in the team. The role may be handed over to the more senior clinicians when they arrive. Leadership can be defined in terms of the attributes of a leader or the process of leadership. Some regard leadership as essential within resuscitation teams. [329, 330] Clearer leadership is associated with more efficient cooperation in the team and also with better task performance.

The team leader should be aware of their own limitations and leadership style (and how this may change during and after the resuscitation scenario according to need [331]). They need to:

- prioritise tasks

- allocate resources and delegate roles clearly

- call for additional help if needed

- moderate and control dialogue

- listen to those around whose input and observations may be invaluable

- reassess regularly and rectify problems

- deal with any conflict (see above)

- maintain a strategic overview of everything and plan ahead.

Just as leadership is important; so too is membership of the team. In some cases staff may be called to a resuscitation and may not know one another, or what skills, background and experience they have. This can make it much more difficult for a potential team leader to give commands and to influence people to follow decisions and work together safely and efficiently. All should be committed to a good patient outcome and should:

- communicate clearly the clinical findings and actions *they* have taken to treat a patient

- be prepared to raise concerns about clinical or safety issues

- endeavour to help the team leader by listening carefully to briefing and instructions and communicating as necessary

- support and show respect for other team members and show tolerance towards hesitancy or nervousness in the emergency setting

- perform skills to the best of their ability

- admit when they cannot do something and need help

- be assertive enough to encourage debate about management if required or draw attention to a problem, but without being destructive

- feel sufficiently empowered to speak out and speak up in presence of errors.

Task management

During any resuscitation there may be a number of tasks which need to be carried out. Effective delegation within the team enables more than one task to be dealt with at the same time enabling faster resolution (Figure 12.1).

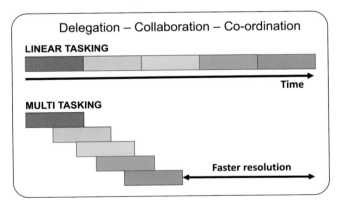

Figure 12.1 The importance of multitasking

The management of a preterm baby after delivery needs prior planning to ensure a coordinated approach:

- Is the baby to be delivered on to the mother's abdomen to allow skin-to-skin?

- Who will deal with the plastic bag and hat?

- Who will assess?

- Who will clamp the cord and transfer to the resuscitaire?

- Who will place the saturation probe on the right wrist?

- Who will manage the airway?

- Is the resuscitaire set up correctly?

- Who will note the time/start the clock/take notes?

- Who will brief/support the parents?

Mistakes will be made and can take many forms – some minor, others potentially catastrophic. Ignorance, assumption, misinterpretation, fixation, coupled to human traits such as arrogance, incompetence, lack of confidence with confounding factors such as suboptimal staffing, excessive workload, etc. Whatever the origin, it is important to recognise their possibility and through effective systems, processes, technical skill and team working minimise their probability, and optimise their identification and rectification. [332, 333]

Communication

Those involved with any resuscitation event need to be able to make decisions, and communicate these effectively. The SBAR tool may help but it is important that within any team, there is a team leader through whom communications are brokered. Any dialogue needs to be precise. Instructions should be directed to specific individuals, with clear identification of the outcome. Where a response is expected, this should be confirmed – the so called 'closed loop'. For example, the person who is managing the airway may say to their colleague "*I am going to give five inflation breaths. Dr Smith, could you please listen to the heart rate and tell me what it is after the fifth breath*". [334]

It is vital that there is mutual respect within a team and that all involved with resuscitation feel able to communicate with each other. Just because someone is a junior member of the team, does not mean that their contribution is invalid. They may have spotted something very important. [335, 336]

The team leader may change as different team members arrive. They may not be the most senior member of the team but it is important that they are clearly identified. Good team leaders need communication, decision-making, organisational and delegating skills. They need to have the knowledge to be able to manage the situation effectively, to be able to recognise if things are going as planned and importantly if they are not, and when extra help is required. [331]

Confidence vs. competence:

The conscious competence learning model (Figure 12.2) suggests that there are four stages to the process and stages of learning a new skill. As people learn they pass

through the four stages:

- learners or trainees tend to begin at stage 1 - 'unconscious incompetence'

- they pass through stage 2 - 'conscious incompetence', then through stage 3 - 'conscious competence'

- and ideally end at stage 4 - 'unconscious competence'.

Do you know where you sit? What about those on your team?

Knowledge of the people you are working with is important when delegating tasks and entrusting responsibility to others. Those who are 'incompetent' need to be watched; the 'confident incompetent' may be a potential hazard - they are a liability. Those who are not confident, but competent need to be supported, and those who are confident and competent relied upon to perform.

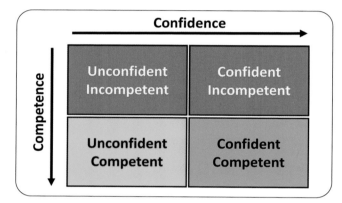

Figure 12.2 The conscious competence learning matrix

The purpose of NLS and many similar training courses is to improve the management of complex situations. Individuals within any group are heterogeneous in their abilities. Prior knowledge of team members can be very helpful in judging their worth in a situation. Personal insight into abilities is also helpful.

Rehearsal

The NLS course was developed to introduce to those involved with babies at birth, a structured, evidence-based approach to newborn life support and an opportunity to begin acquisition of the psychomotor and team working skills required to apply the algorithm effectively to a variety of situations. It enables individuals to refine both their individual skills and their approach within a team. The NLS course is an ideal time to make mistakes, to practice a new approach and observe how others deal with difficult situations so that once back in the clinical area performance and outcomes are improved.

Whilst practice through workshops and simulations may not equate to the 'real thing' they nevertheless permit the practice of the psychomotor skills, sequencing and team working even if the actual procedures are carried out on plastic manikins which are not like the real thing.

Although the NLS course begins the process of good practice it is clear from the literature documenting skill retention after adult learning, and best practice in clinical simulation, that it is the responsibility of any individual who becomes an NLS provider to continue to practice the skills and team working taught on the course in their own clinical environment. [337] For those in busy units this will involve regular application of the skills in real life. Those in less busy or low-risk environments (e.g. stand-alone midwife led units or community settings) will have to ensure they engage in regular manikin simulation sessions in order to maintain proficiency. If no regular application of the skills learned occurs, the provider will de-skill regardless of having previously attained the standard required to pass the course.

Debrief

It is important to be able to reflect on performance. Following any resuscitation or simulation practice it should be a priority to ensure that team members have the opportunity to review events and discuss any issues. Ideally such debriefs need to involve all team members and take place as soon after the event as possible. They need to be non-judgemental, but constructive in how issues are dealt with. They may be facilitated by staff who were not involved, or just involve those who attended. Where someone is facilitating a learning debrief following a simulation practice, they should ideally have been in a purely observational role whilst the simulation was on-going. Those debriefing should have experience and training in how to undertake this. Through immediate debrief it may be possible to identify areas of good or suboptimal performance which can then feed back into the management of future resuscitations. [338-340] Through the identification of potential problems it improves governance and ensures matters are dealt with in a timely and appropriate manner.

Summary learning

- **Prior planning of the approach to resuscitation makes success more likely.**

- **Knowledge of processes involved, ability to undertake procedures and awareness of the dynamics of team working are important in the optimal management of any resuscitation.**

- **Clear and reliable lines of communication are vital.**

- **Rehearsal of and debrief following resuscitation situations enhance learning and improve future management.**

My key take-home messages from this chapter

A cautionary note, controversies, and other miscellanea

Contents

- **Cord clamping**
- **Cord "milking" or "stripping"**
- **Use of CPAP and/or PEEP at birth**
- **The approach to the baby born through meconium-stained amniotic fluid**
- **Chest compressions – different ventilation:compression ratios**
- **Sodium bicarbonate**
- **Intratracheal adrenaline**
- **Naloxone and maternal opiate abuse**
- **'Sustained' inflations**
- **Can cord gases tell us when a hypoxic insult began?**
- **The Apgar score**
- **Sarnat grading (Sarnat score)**

Learning outcomes

To enable you to:

- **Appreciate that not everything is known about newborn resuscitation**
- **Understand where uncertainties exist and how these are being addressed in a pragmatic way**

A cautionary note

This manual is a consensus statement and one should always be sceptical of such statements. Just because everyone agrees you should do something a particular way does not mean that that really is the best way to do it. We would do well to remember the words of Sir Thomas Clifford Allbutt (1836–1925), English physician and inventor of the clinical thermometer:

> "*our path is cumbered with guesses, presumptions and conjectures, the untimely and sterile fruitage of minds which cannot wait for the facts, and are ready to forget that the use of hypothesis lies not in the display of ingenuity but in the labour of verification*". [341]

There are many controversies in the field of neonatal resuscitation and little strong experimental evidence is currently available to resolve them. Publication of an opinion, even in a highly reputable journal, does not mean that that opinion is correct. In 1951 a leading article in the Lancet entitled "Anoxia in the Newborn" confidently stated that "*any method of attempting pulmonary expansion by blowing gases into the trachea under pressure must be condemned*". [309] We now know that this is not only safe, but in certain circumstances it is a highly desirable practice.

In the 1960s respiratory stimulants were commonly used but we now know them to be both ineffective and potentially dangerous. Even in the 21st century many experts strongly recommended that the nose and mouth of the baby should be aspirated before the shoulders were delivered in labours complicated by meconium-stained liquor. However, since 2004 we have known from a large multi-centre randomised controlled study that such intrapartum suctioning is not effective in preventing meconium aspiration syndrome. [157] We have also learnt that routine suctioning of the airway of *any* baby born through meconium stained liquor is not only ineffective, but also potentially injurious, especially to those screaming babies whose airways were clearly patent. [158, 342-344] Latterly we have learnt that routinely suctioning the trachea of even the floppiest of these babies may not be as effective as once thought, and that spending time removing meconium may delay the onset of basic resuscitation. [345]

Many other examples of ineffective treatments exist. Future work will hopefully resolve some of these controversies but others will certainly arise to take their place.

Much of the physiological evidence on which the strategies of neonatal resuscitation are based relates to sudden total anoxia. In real life intermittent partial hypoxia of varying severity, frequency and duration, with or without accompanying ischaemia, is the more common pattern of intrapartum insult that the fetus has to face. The physiological response to this pattern of stresses is less well explored and may be subtly different. Furthermore, the response of a chronically stressed baby whose intrauterine growth has been compromised may well be different to that of a well grown baby facing significant problems for the first time. Heart rate responses to stress in labour differ between male and female babies. It is also likely that the quality and nature of any fetal responses will vary with varying degrees of fetal maturity.

While the current enthusiasm for detailed protocols continues it should be remembered that a protocol is only as good as the experimental evidence on which it is based. The advice in this manual constitutes a guide to resuscitation at birth, not a protocol. It represents the collective opinion of many with extensive personal experience of performing neonatal resuscitation as well as teaching the subject. The advice given does not define the **only** way that resuscitation at birth should be performed. We merely suggest that it is an accepted view of how resuscitation at birth can be carried out both safely and effectively.

Controversies

When considering the practicalities of newborn resuscitation one encounters a number of controversial areas. Most of these are capable of generating an amount of heated argument quite out of proportion to their importance. Nevertheless these controversies still cause distress, confusion and debate and some controversies are of greater potential importance. This section will attempt to set out some of the evidence on either side of the various debates and put the arguments in context.

When should the umbilical cord be clamped?

This question has been asked in various forms for at least 200 years and the issue is now being debated once again. So-called 'active management of the third stage of labour' was introduced in the 1970s primarily to address the problem of post-partum haemorrhage. Such active management involves giving an intramuscular injection of syntometrine to the mother immediately after emergence of the baby, with the cord usually being clamped before the injection was given. Little thought appears to have been given to any effect on the baby.

There have been a number of studies comparing 'early' versus so-called 'delayed' clamping of the cord. The definition of what constitutes 'early' clamping varies between 'immediate', less than 20 s, less than 1 min and, in the early literature, less than 5 min. The definition of late clamping has been similarly variable.

Clamping of the cord before the baby has taken a breath is associated with a drop in heart rate that is not seen if clamping occurs after the first breath. [346] When viewed on video-radiography, a decrease in heart size for three or four cardiac cycles is seen if clamping occurs before the first breath. [347] One suggested reason for this is that the increased cardiac output necessary to begin filling the pulmonary circulation, which normally occurs with the first few breaths, is easily replenished from the placenta via the umbilical circulation if the cord is unclamped. If this is the correct explanation then clearly this rapid replenishment cannot occur if breathing does not start until after the cord is clamped. Venous return to the heart is then temporarily inadequate for a few beats until blood begins to return from the lungs into the left atrium. Studies of placental transfusion rate and uterine contraction failed to show any clear relationship between infant blood volume in the first hour of life and timing of cord clamping in relation to establishment of regular respiration. [348]

How the total volume of blood in the conceptus is distributed between the placenta and the baby can change during labour and at delivery. Furthermore, pressure on the cord, such as might occlude the soft-walled umbilical vein but fail to occlude the muscular-walled umbilical arteries, has been held to be responsible for neonatal hypovolaemia sufficient to cause shock. [349]

There are also concerns that a similar process whereby pressure on the fetal thorax in the birth canal during obstructed labour, for example in shoulder dystocia, may transfer a significant volume of blood from the compressed fetus to the placenta. If the cord is then clamped and cut before the compression is relieved by the birth of the baby, then this blood cannot return from the placenta, which might leave the baby seriously hypovolaemic. [350]

Delayed clamping of the cord in babies who are born at term is associated with a better iron status during the first few months, presumably because it allows a greater placenta tranfusion to the baby after delivery. An increase in clinical jaundice and use of phototherapy has been reported in various studies but this is perhaps less worrying than it first appears given that the criteria for the use of phototherapy were neither defined nor controlled and more invasive treatment of jaundice was apparently not required.

In preterm infants the observed benefits of later clamping are greater stability during the immediate postnatal transition, more stable blood pressure, reduced use of pressor agents and a reduced perceived necessity for early or later transfusion. [4, 243, 244, 351] Also, waiting before clamping the cord might conceivably increase the passage of stem cells to the baby. [352] Concerns about increased jaundice, unintentional hypothermia, increased need for exchange transfusion for hyperbilirubinaemia (or polycythaemia), or increased respiratory distress have not been confirmed. [244]

Unfortunately babies apparently needing significant resuscitation were excluded from all these studies so it is not possible to say with any certainty whether later cord clamping is appropriate under those circumstances. Furthermore, the physiological animal studies described in Chapter four were all performed with the umbilical cord occluded at the onset of the hypoxic insult and later divided. Any effect of re-establishing the feto-placental circulation in the treatment of the hypoxic insult was therefore not explored.

It should perhaps be remembered that, although it may be more **convenient** to transfer the baby to a resuscitaire to provide resuscitation such transfer is not an essential feature of resuscitation itself. Indeed, if the placenta has not separated from the uterine wall, it may even be advantageous to the baby to start resuscitation without clamping or cutting the cord. [353]

The 2012 World Health Organisation recommendations for the prevention and treatment of postpartum haemorrhage, state:

"Late cord clamping (performed after 1 to 3 minutes after birth) is recommended for all births while initiating simultaneous essential newborn care. (Strong recommendation, moderate quality evidence).

Early cord clamping (<1 minute after birth) is not recommended unless the neonate is asphyxiated and needs to be moved immediately for resuscitation. (Strong recommendation, moderate-quality evidence)." [354]

In 2014, the National Institute for Health and Care Excellence (NICE) guideline for intrapartum care states *"Do not clamp the cord earlier than 1 minute from the birth of the baby unless there is concern about the integrity of the cord or the baby has a heartbeat below 60*

beats/minute that is not getting faster". [272] This follows the 2009 Royal College of Obstetricians and Gynaecologists Scientific Advisory Committee opinion entitled 'Clamping of the umbilical cord and placental transfusion' [355] which acknowledged that *"for decades immediate cord clamping has been bundled into the package of care known as 'active management' and the potential consequences either ignored or forgotten".* They also strongly support further investigation of this issue by mean of large randomised controlled trials.

In 2010 the International Liaison Committee on Resuscitation (ILCOR) considered the published evidence and issued the following recommendation: *"Delay in umbilical cord clamping for at least 1 minute is recommended for newborn infants not requiring resuscitation. There is insufficient evidence to support or refute a recommendation to delay cord clamping in babies requiring resuscitation."* [356, 357] In the preamble to this recommendation they stated *"There are limited data on the hazards or benefits of delayed cord clamping in the non-vigorous infant".*

In 2015 the debate centred on cord clamping in preterm babies who **required resuscitation**. After consideration of the evidence, which the neonatal ILCOR group felt was of low quality and thus downgraded for imprecision and very high risk of bias, it was not felt possible to provide a definitive answer in this scenario. The recommendations state:

*"We **suggest** delayed umbilical cord clamping for preterm infants not requiring immediate resuscitation after birth. (Weak recommendation, very low quality of evidence)*

There is insufficient evidence to recommend an approach to cord clamping for preterm infants who do receive resuscitation immediately after birth, as many babies who were at high risk of requiring resuscitation were excluded from or withdrawn from the studies." [17, 18]

Whilst much evidence is pointing in the direction of delayed cord clamping, many questions remain unanswered: What should drive clamping of the cord? Should it wait until the baby takes a spontaneous breath, or until cord pulsation has ceased, or should it wait a specific length of time: if this last, then what length of time is appropriate and might that time differ following delivery by section or if blood in the cord was 'milked' towards the baby before clamping? Is this pause affected by the timing, dose or route of administration of uterotonics? Should this pause also occur if the baby has no detectable heart rate at delivery or should one consider milking the cord before clamping in this situation? Should the cord be clamped before providing positive pressure ventilation? Should the same instructions apply to all babies – including both those apparently needing resuscitation and those born very preterm?

Good quality randomised controlled trials are urgently needed to address questions such as these and such trials should involve all babies, including those apparently needing resuscitation and the very preterm. Perinatal consequences of early and later clamping to both the mother and the baby need to be evaluated in these trials and neuro-developmental outcomes should also be compared, particularly in relation to preterm babies.

Is milking ('stripping') the umbilical cord a viable alternative to delayed cord clamping?

The increasing evidence that placental transfusion after delayed cord clamping is beneficial in healthy babies not requiring resuscitation has, understandably, led to the question how to address this issue in the babies that **do** require resuscitation.

In some cases a delay in clamping and cutting the cord may compromise either the mother or the baby; a delay might interfere with management of maternal haemorrhage, very low birth weight babies might develop hypothermia due to the difficulties with thermal protection while the cord is still attached. In most cases, the design and equipment of delivery centres do not allow for the resuscitation of infants before placenta separation and so, in almost all cases, the default position in the compromised baby becomes early cord clamping.

Umbilical cord 'milking' or 'stripping' has been proposed as an alternative to delayed cord clamping when the baby or the mother may be harmed by that delay. Cord milking involves rapid transfer of blood from the placenta towards the baby and actively moves blood from the cord and placenta to the baby. Milking of the cord can be completed in around 20 s [358], much shorter than the 30–180 s recommended with delayed clamping of the cord.

Uncontrolled studies have shown that cord milking can be beneficial; more blood flows through the lungs [359], and cardiovascular stability is improved in both preterm and term babies [360-362]. There are also studies that have shown milking can have a detrimental effect; cord milking can increase the baby's blood volume by up to 22% and red cell volume by 45%. [363] Over-enthusiastic milking (10 times over a 5 min period) was reported to be responsible for one baby becoming cyanosed and requiring admission to the neonatal unit. [358] More contemporary studies milking a segment (typically of 20 cm length) of cord rapidly 3–5 times have not reported any such adverse events. [358-362, 364, 365]

Many of these studies were considered during the 2015 ILCOR deliberations which concluded that there was insufficient published evidence of benefit to recommend this procedure routinely, but that it "*may be considered on an individualized basis or in a research setting as it may improve initial mean blood pressure, haematological*

indices and intracranial haemorrhage". [17] Both the ILCOR recommendations and a meta-analysis [248] of this procedure caution that there are few data on neonatal and long-term outcomes. It would follow that the technique described in the contemporary studies should be the one used in these situations and that at present there are few data to support this over delayed cord clamping in healthy babies of any gestation.

Use of CPAP and/or PEEP at birth

When attending the delivery of preterm infants, one is more commonly involved in stabilisation ('assisted transition') of a fragile infant rather than resuscitation of a nearly dead one. In the absence of good evidence to act differently one might reasonably suppose that gentle support of spontaneous respiration, with CPAP alone, rather than immediate intubation, might have advantages.

Continuous positive airway pressure or CPAP has been around since the 1950s but has attracted renewed interest in the past 15–20 years. A randomised controlled trial in preterm lambs has shown that the group receiving CPAP had higher lung volumes and less histological evidence of inflammation than a comparison group who were ventilated from birth. [366] Use of PEEP from the outset in the ventilation of newborn animals has been shown to reduce the amount of lung inflammation and to preserve surfactant function in preterm animal models. [367] In a historic cohort study transitional support with a bag and mask and stabilization of extremely low birth weight (ELBW) infants on CPAP resulted in a quarter of them never being intubated. [11]

Early reservations about this strategy centred on the fact that early application of CPAP with the intention of avoiding intubation would deprive the baby of the advantages of early ('prophylactic') compared to later ('rescue') administration of surfactant supplementation. There are now three large randomised trials that examine the strategy of initial stabilisation on nasal CPAP versus conventional management of intubation and surfactant administration in preterm infants; the CPAP Or nasal INtubation at birth (COIN) trial [259], the Surfactant Positive Pressure and Oxygen Randomized Trial (SUPPORT) [368] and the Vermont Oxford Network Delivery Room Management (VON DRM) trial [369]. These and several smaller trials were included in a Cochrane meta-analysis that concludes that, with the routine use of CPAP in babies at risk of developing RDS, "*the benefits of prophylactic surfactant could no longer be demonstrated*". [370]

There is, therefore, good evidence for the use of CPAP or PEEP in the preterm infant, this facilitates lung aeration and maintains lung volume. It does mean, however, that these infants are best managed with a T-piece device, not a self-inflating or flow-inflating bag. Self-inflating bags cannot deliver positive end-expiratory pressure (PEEP) and so are not ideal for helping to form and maintain the functional residual capacity (FRC) in a very preterm baby. A PEEP valve can be fitted but the pressure is not constant, moreover, PEEP can only be provided if the bag is squeezed at least 40 times per minute and even then level of PEEP will vary with the rate. [142]

The evidence for use of PEEP in those term infants that require positive pressure ventilation during resuscitation is less clear, and the ILCOR neonatal group were unable to make any recommendation for term infants because of insufficient data. [17] In theory, at least, use of PEEP in this group would seem a good idea, spontaneously breathing newborn babies commonly make expiratory braking manoeuvres that help to maintain FRC by extending the expiratory flow time and increasing airway pressure during passive expiration. [371, 372] These manoeuvres only seem to occur after an FRC has been established, but they do appear to be mostly associated with maintaining that FRC.

The approach to the baby born through meconium-stained amniotic fluid

The management of the baby born through meconium-stained liquor has changed markedly in the past 50 years. The 1960s and 1970s saw the emergence of several management strategies that have since been examined more closely in large randomised controlled trails and been found to be ineffective. Chief among these was to routinely suction the nose and mouth of the baby whilst the head was 'on the perineum' [373] and to intubate the infant as soon as possible after delivery [374]. Before 1975, few babies were either suctioned by midwives and obstetricians and few were intubated by paediatricians, but by the end of that decade, the standard of care was changed to include routine intubation and tracheal suctioning of all babies born through meconium-stained liquor. [375] Some groups even advocated compressing the chest post-delivery until the trachea could be intubated. [376]

All this was undertaken in the mistaken belief that inhalation of the meconium occurred after delivery and that if the upper airways and trachea were cleared then aspiration could not occur. Such was the belief in this approach that even as late as 1990 papers were being published that stated "*the decline in MAS* (meconium aspiration syndrome) *is primarily due to routine oropharyngeal suctioning by obstetricians and subsequent postpartum intratracheal suctioning.*" [377] Babies were therefore subjected to repeated intubations and tracheal suction until such time that the fluid returned was not meconium-stained [378], and presumably often deteriorating further during such suctioning.

We now know that most babies born through meconium-stained liquor have not inhaled any particulate material into the lower respiratory tract and if they have not done so as a result of anoxic gasping before birth they will only very rarely do so at birth. [113] Large, multi-centre randomised studies were published in full in 2000 and 2004 that showed that the previously advocated practices of aspirating the airways of the emerging baby before delivery followed by intubation and suction of the trachea after

delivery – the so-called '*combined obstetric and paediatric approach*' – was not effective and did not prevent the development of meconium aspiration syndrome. [157, 158] Moreover there was increasing evidence suggesting that attempting to inspect the oropharynx or even intubate vigorous term babies was harmful. [379] Accordingly since 2000 newborn resuscitation guidelines have advised that suction of the upper airways when the head was delivered was of no benefit, but continued to advocate that the depressed (i.e. floppy) baby must be intubated and suctioned if the resuscitator was skilled at intubation. [380]

The 2015 guidance goes one step further and the ILCOR neonatal deliberations concluded that there is "*insufficient published human evidence to suggest routine tracheal intubation for suctioning of meconium in non-vigorous infants born through meconium-stained amniotic fluid as opposed to no tracheal intubation for suctioning*" and instead advocates minimising the delay in starting positive pressure ventilation within the first minute of life. [17] A recently published randomised trial [114] along with a similar study performed in India and presented at the 2014 Pediatric Academic Societies meeting (and thus available in abstract only) [155] showed no differences in any reported clinical outcomes whether babies were intubated or not.

With these studies in mind the ILCOR neonatal group recommended that "*routine tracheal intubation for suctioning of meconium in non-vigorous infants should not be considered as a standard of care but may be considered.....if tracheal obstruction is suspected*". [17] In interpreting these recommendations we have therefore stated that;

> "*If a baby born through meconium-stained amniotic fluid is also floppy and makes no immediate respiratory effort, then it is probably reasonable to rapidly inspect the oropharynx with a view to removing any particulate matter that might obstruct the airway. However, in a bradycardic baby the emphasis must be to inflate the lungs within the first minute after birth and this must not be delayed. There is no evidence to support routine tracheal suctioning in this situation unless there is evidence that the trachea is blocked.*"

In other words, if you are able to do so you can rapidly inspect the oropharynx, spending as little time as possible suctioning, before moving on to inflating the lungs. If you cannot inflate the lungs consider the possibility that the trachea may be blocked and that it may be necessary to intubate the trachea to remove any meconium. If you cannot intubate, then you should not delay inflating the lungs pending the arrival of someone who can intubate; consider using higher inflation pressures or longer breaths.

Chest compressions

Chest compressions when used in resuscitation may be administered in a number of different ways, in a variety of ratios and may (or may not) be synchronised with ventilation breaths. Until recently the ways in which chest compressions are delivered were poorly researched and evidence still remains sparse.

NLS

When to switch from the newborn 3:1 to the paediatric 15:2 compressions to ventilation ratio

A major difference between the newborn and paediatric guidelines is in the ratio of compressions to ventilations in CPR. The ILCOR evaluation of the evidence for these two groups arrived at different conclusions. Newborn babies and those on medical neonatal units, special care units and postnatal wards should usually receive 3 compressions to 1 ventilation as the reason for resuscitation is most likely to be respiratory and this ratio is most likely to deliver an appropriate ventilation rate. If a baby is thought to have a primary cardiac cause for arrest consideration should be given to using a ratio of 15 compressions to 2 ventilations.

A baby who has successfully adapted to extra-uterine life and has subsequently collapsed and presented to the emergency department, or collapsed on a joint neonatal/paediatric medical and surgical intensive care unit should be resuscitated according to paediatric life support algorithms with a 15:2 compression to ventilation ratio.

Sodium bicarbonate

This manual recommends that drugs should **only** be used in those very rare situations where the heart rate has not responded to adequate lung aeration, ventilation and chest compressions. Some, however, have significant reservations about using bicarbonate. [381, 382] On closer inspection these reservations relate to the practice of rapidly correcting acidosis following resuscitation or infusion of bicarbonate routinely during resuscitation – reservations which are reasonable. [383] However, it does not follow that bicarbonate should be disregarded altogether.

Good quality evidence for or against the use of sodium bicarbonate in human newborns who are severely compromised due to hypoxia is sadly lacking. Only one small (under-powered) randomised trial in human newborn resuscitation, reported in two separate publications [384, 385], has looked at the effects of sodium bicarbonate in affected newborn babies. This study randomly allocated babies who were still receiving positive pressure ventilation at 5 min of age to treatment with sodium bicarbonate (n=27) or a dextrose placebo (n=28). The investigators concluded bicarbonate does not help to improve survival or immediate neurological outcome. There are some issues with the study; that only 12 of the group treated with bicarbonate (and 11 of the placebo group) received chest compressions throws an element of doubt into the validity of the study in its extrapolation to the situation of an asystolic newborn where drugs are currently advocated only after chest compressions have been shown to be ineffective. In addition, the mean Apgar scores at one minute and at five minutes were lower, more babies were born through meconium-stained liquor and more babies were given adrenaline in the bicarbonate

group suggesting that the two groups were not as well matched as they might have been.

Some of the early work on animals examined the effect of injecting either respiratory stimulants or base intravenously, in these studies the alkali used was the organic base, trometamol (formerly better known as tris-hydroxymethyl-aminomethane or THAM) rather than bicarbonate. These animals (fetal monkeys) were known to have taken their last gasp and thus known to be in terminal apnoea. [79] The injection of the respiratory stimulants lobeline or nikethamide resulted in a fall in blood pressure whereas the injection of THAM (0.5% molar solution with 3.5% dextrose, with the pH adjusted to 8.85) caused a rise in both heart rate and blood pressure and the recurrence of gasping allowing the monkeys to be successfully resuscitated using positive pressure ventilation.

This is why this text would like to be able to continue to recommend that sodium bicarbonate be considered if adequate lung aeration, ventilation and chest compression achieve no increase in heart rate.

Unfortunately, the effect of adrenaline was not investigated in the experiment described in the previous paragraph. Animal data shows that the binding of adrenaline to its receptors in the myocardium is significantly impaired by lactic acidosis [386] and studies on human lymphocyte beta-adrenergic receptors supports this view [226]. Whether this is also true of the more important alpha receptors is unknown.

Intratracheal adrenaline

In order to overcome some of the delay associated with intravenous administration of adrenaline at newborn resuscitation it has been suggested that adrenaline can be effective when given down the tracheal tube into the lungs. [225] Few of the animal studies of this technique have been done in newborn animals whose lungs have just been aerated. It appears to be effective in adult (human) resuscitation provided a dose of at least 2 mg of adrenaline is given. [387] However, a study using newborn piglets suggests that while doses given intravenously had measurable effects on carotid blood pressure, similar doses given via the tracheal tube do not. [388] Evidence from one case series showed response was more common after intravenous adrenaline than after a similar dose of tracheal adrenaline. [389] This is consistent with evidence extrapolated from neonatal animal models indicating that higher doses (50–100 microgram kg^{-1}) of tracheal adrenaline may be required to achieve the increased blood adrenaline concentrations and haemodynamic responses seen after intravenous administration. [390, 391] Although it has been widely assumed that adrenaline can be administered faster by the tracheal route than the intravenous route, no clinical trials have evaluated this hypothesis. Whether effective or not, if you want to give tracheal adrenaline then a tracheal tube needs to be in place.

Naloxone and maternal opiate abuse

Many guidelines on resuscitation at birth warn against giving naloxone to the baby of an opiate abusing mother for fear of inducing fits. As justification all quote the same single brief case report of fits in a newborn baby that was attributed to this cause. [392] In this report, seizures are reported to have started two minutes after the baby received a 200 microgram intramuscular dose of naloxone shortly after birth, and to have stopped thirty minutes later just as soon as a 100 microgram kg^{-1} bolus of morphine was given intravenously. There are, for many people, additional details that are missing from the report; the baby was delivered by caesarean section for "fetal distress" although the nature of this is not given; there were no umbilical cord gases stated; the baby only received naloxone after failing to breath spontaneously at four minutes of age (suggesting that the respiratory depression may have been caused by the very "fetal distress" that led to the section in the first place).

This remains, after twenty five years, the only published report of such a complication and, since no other case has ever been reported to the UK or other licensing authorities. That said, the use of naloxone has declined substantially since the report was published and there has been a general move away from naloxone use as a "drug of resuscitation". These changes, alone, might explain the absence of any further reports through any pharmacovigilance schemes such as the Medicines and Healthcare products Regulatory Agency's yellow card scheme. There are, nonetheless, anecdotal reports of acute opiate withdrawal symptoms in babies whose mothers have been taking opiates and where the baby was given naloxone shortly after birth. The withdrawal symptoms involved agitation and jitteriness and started in the delivery room, none, however, have been seizures.

It is probable that the infant of a mother who has been regularly abusing opiates during pregnancy is less likely to have respiratory depression from maternal opiates given in labour than an infant whose mother had not used opiates before.

Intraosseous access

There is no evidence for the effectiveness or otherwise of intraosseous infusion of drugs in resuscitation at birth. Recent data suggest that the intraosseous route can be effective in the resuscitation of preterm and full term infants in the intensive care unit when alternative venous access proves impossible to establish. [221] However, it is difficult to justify the insertion of such a device into the bone of a newborn baby when umbilical venous catheterisation so easily provides central venous access of known efficacy.

The technique should perhaps be reserved for those extremely rare occasions when a baby requiring resuscitation at birth also has a problem, such as exomphalos, which makes umbilical venous catheterisation

more difficult. [393-395] The other situation where it might be useful is in resuscitation outside labour ward (e.g. in the Emergency Department) where staff are more familiar with the intraosseus needle insertion technique. [222]

'Sustained' inflations

The Newborn Life Support course has long advocated the use of what it calls "inflation breaths", using the term to describe the 2–3 s aeration breaths given at the start of resuscitation. Early work describing the first breaths of life in normal full term babies had shown them to be characterised by prolonged expiratory phases, associated with high positive intrathoracic pressure, interspersed with brief inspiratory components. The investigators therefore postulated that the phase of high positive pressure may facilitate the distribution of air within the lungs and assist in the formation of the functional residual capacity (FRC). [396] During studies of sustained lung inflation in the resuscitation of compromised hypoxic babies it was shown that a large increase in the tidal volume and the FRC could be achieved with sustained inflations. [116]

The inflation breaths described in this manual (and its predecessors) are not to be confused with 'sustained inflation' breaths used in studies considered by the 2015 neonatal ILCOR group. [17] The group asked whether in non-breathing term or preterm newborn infants "*does administration of one or more pressure-limited sustained lung inflations, compared to intermittent PPV with short inspiratory times improve outcomes*" and considered evidence from a number of trials where the duration of such inflation breaths ranged from 5 s to 20 s. [119, 397-399] In addition, there were some studies that had co-interventions that limited any direct comparisons.

After consideration of the evidence the ILCOR neonatal group decided to "*suggest against the routine use of initial sustained inflation (>5 seconds duration) for preterm infants without spontaneous respirations immediately after birth*". Further studies, however, are needed before this strategy may be fully discounted; a recent meta-analysis that included those trials considered by the ILCOR neonatal group showed that infants who received sustained lung inflations spent less time on a ventilator. [400]

For the time being, the NLS course will continue to use the term "inflation breaths" for the 2–3 s duration aeration breaths at the start of resuscitation but cannot recommend "sustained inflations" of >5 s duration unless this is within the context of a properly conducted clinical trial.

Can cord gases tell us when the hypoxic insult began?

If there are concerns that the baby has been significantly compromised it can be helpful to obtain blood for measurement of pH, base deficit and lactate both from an umbilical artery as well as from the vein. [290-293]

	ARTERIAL		VENOUS	
	Mean (± 1SD)	Range	Mean (± 1SD)	Range
pH	7.28 (± 0.05)	7.15–7.43	7.35 (± 0.05)	7.24–7.49
PCO_2 (kPa)	6.56 (± 1.12)	4.15–9.91	5.09 (± 0.75)	3.09–6.56
PO_2 (kPa)	2.40 (± 0.83)	0.51–4.51	3.89 (± 0.79)	2.05–6.42
Bicarbonate (mmol/L)	22.3 (± 2.5)	13.3–27.5	20.4 (± 2.1)	15.9–24.7

Table A1.1 Normal ranges for blood gas parameters from umbilical artery and venous samples from uncomplicated vaginal deliveries

Whilst the results of these do not usually impact on the resuscitation (usually the result is not known until after the resuscitation is finished), they can nonetheless provide some useful information about the gas exchange processes in the minutes leading up to delivery. The analyses must, however, be done in a timely fashion. [290]

If paired arterial and venous samples are obtained it is the arterial sample that shows a lower pH, higher carbon dioxide and lactate and a worse base excess (this is different from the usual situation where venous blood gases are worse). This is because the umbilical *arterial* gases reflect the status of the fetus, whereas the umbilical *venous* gases reflect the ability of the placenta to deal with the excess carbon dioxide and lactic acid from the fetus. The range of 'normal values' from 146 uncomplicated vaginal deliveries at term [401] is shown in Table A1.1.

In general, the lower range for normal arterial pH extends to at least 7.10 and that for venous pH to at least 7.20. There is no consensus as to what constitutes significant acidosis; the pH values that have been used to define acidosis range from 7.20 to 7.00. [402, 403] There is a poor relationship between Apgar score, need for resuscitation and eventual neurodevelopmental outcome and cord pH; whilst only 2% of babies with a normal Apgar score have a pH <7.10, most babies with a cord blood pH between 7.00 and 7.10 will have a normal Apgar score. It is only when the cord blood pH reaches levels less than 7.00 that low Apgar scores become common. [403]

In an acutely and continuously compromised fetus where placental gas exchange is compromised, there is a progressive fall in pH from 7.32 to 7.00 at 5 min and to 6.8 at 10 min. [404] Once severe acidosis is present, the likelihood of adverse sequelae rises sharply with worsening acidosis; the numbers of infants with hypoxic-ischaemic encephalopathy increased steadily with worsening cord pH from 12% with cord pH <7.0, 33% with cord pH <6.9, 60% with cord pH <6.8, and 80% with cord pH <6.7. [405] No infants survived when the cord pH was <6.6. [405]

When paired venous and arterial umbilical cord samples are taken it is possible to get some indication of the timing of the hypoxic insult in terms of it being 'acute' or 'chronic'. This is because the fetus produces carbon dioxide and lactic acid, both of which are removed by the placenta. Most cases of fetal acidosis during labour are acute in onset, and in most cases the placenta retains the ability to compensate for much of the excess acids produced by the hypoxic fetus. However if the insult is profound and prolonged, then this compensatory mechanism is over-whelmed. Thus a 'bad' umbilical arterial gas paired with a 'better' venous gas is suggestive of a more recent event, whereas if both arterial and venous samples are bad then the event is more likely to have been more prolonged. [292]

Other factors, however, come into play and the cord blood gases should not be viewed in isolation. Differences between arterial and venous samples may be pronounced in nuchal cords (i.e. when the umbilical cord becomes wrapped at least once around the fetal neck) [406] and reduced when there is placental abruption [407]. If the insult was a cord obstruction that is released shortly before delivery it is possible that the umbilical arterial and venous gases can be normal despite severe intrapartum compromise and even fetal demise. [293, 408]

Umbilical cord gases provide a useful indication of the extent of compromise in many cases, however they cannot, in isolation, be used to determine the timing of the hypoxic insult. Additional information about the antenatal health of both the mother and the fetus, as well as information about events during labour must be taken into account.

Apgar score			
Score	0	1	2
Colour	Pale/blue	Body pink, extremities blue	Pink
Heart rate	Absent	Less than 100	More than 100
Response to stimulation	Nil	Some movement	Cry
Muscle tone	Limp	Some flexion of extremities	Well flexed
Respiratory effort	Absent	Weak cry or hypoventilation	Good

Table A1.2 The Apgar score is calculated by assigning scores of 0–2 to five physiological and behavioural observations. Resulting in an overall score of 0–10

Scoring systems

The Apgar score and Sarnat grading are common scoring systems used to classify babies at birth or soon after. Sarnat grading is used to grade encephalopathy, particularly if therapeutic hypothermia is being considered. Neither score should be recorded simply as a number. A detailed description of the baby is essential.

The Apgar score

The Apgar score, calculated by assigning scores to various physiological parameters (Table A1.2), has major limitations. It was originally devised for use as *"a basis for discussion and comparison of the results of obstetric practices, types of maternal pain relief and the effects of resuscitation"*. [104] It is of some use in categorising groups of babies, but of no use in the clinical management of individual babies. [409] Virginia Apgar, who was an obstetric anaesthetist, did not expect the score to predict mortality in individual babies but she did hope it might reveal a relationship between condition at birth and long-term neurological outcome. [409] In fact it does do this to some extent but it is very non-specific.

A large cohort study from Norway showed that babies with a very low Apgar score (≤3 at five min) have a 11% risk of showing signs of cerebral palsy (if they survive to one year) as compared with a risk of 0.1% for babies with a very high score (nine or more). [410] However, this tells us little about the cause of the cerebral palsy. Babies with low scores would include those with a longstanding problem prior to birth, those who had suffered a recent adverse event before birth as well as those who suffered an insult during birth. Furthermore this study did not separately analyse the one subset of cerebral palsy most convincingly associated with perinatal hypoxia and subsequent encephalopathy, namely athetoid / dyskinetic cerebral palsy. The study also showed that almost 90% of survivors with a very low score did not have cerebral palsy and 80% of those with cerebral palsy had an Apgar score of seven or more. This agrees well with an American study which showed that 80% of survivors with a score of three or less were entirely normal at school age. [411]

Virginia Apgar certainly drew attention to features which are important in assessing condition at birth but assigning scores to these features seems to have been much less helpful. The respiratory and heart rate scores are more important than the other items and the total score on its own is particularly uninformative. When one considers that each of the five components of the score is a separate ordinal variable it is perhaps not surprising that adding them together (a mathematically inappropriate manoeuvre for this level of measurement) is unhelpful. [412]

While it has long been assumed that a close relationship exists between the Apgar score and pH and umbilical blood gas status at birth, Sykes *et al* showed that this is not so. [413] Only 21% of babies with a one minute Apgar score <7, and 19% of babies with a five minute score <7 had an umbilical artery blood pH <7.1. Conversely 73% with severe acidosis had a one minute ≥7, while 86% had a five minute score ≥7.

In practice the Apgar score is usually recorded retrospectively and subjectively. For these reasons it may be highly unreliable. Many hospitals have never recorded this score and a number of others no longer do so. If it is your practice to record the Apgar score, a written description of all the characteristics used to assign the score must also be recorded as well as the details of any resuscitation.

Sarnat grading (Sarnat score)

In a baby who receives significant resuscitation at birth and who goes on to show signs of encephalopathy it is important to document the neurological state regularly over the first few days and not just at birth. The most useful system for this purpose is the Sarnat grading (Table A1.3). [414] An assessment at 24–48 h gives a much better indication of the long-term prognosis that any permutation of the one, five and 10 min Apgar score. [415]

Sarnat grade			
Grade	**1**	**2**	**3**
Conscious level	Hyperalert	Lethargic or obtunded	Stuporous or comatose
Muscle tone	Normal	Mild hypotonia	Flaccid
Posture	Mild distal flexion	Strong distal flexion	Intermittent decerebration
Stretch reflexes	Overactive	Overactive	Decreased or absent
Moro reflex	Strong	Incomplete	Absent
Suck reflex	Normal	Weak or absent	Absent
Tonic neck reflex	Slight	Strong	Absent
Pupils	Dilated	Constricted	Poorly reactive
Gut motility	Normal	Increased	Variable
Seizures	Uncommon	Focal or multifocal	Mostly decerebrate

Table A1.3 The Sarnat score for evaluating babies with suspected hypoxic-ischaemic brain injury based upon their neurologic features

Early seizures (before 48 hours) are worrying, but signs of a moderate or severe encephalopathy at 24–48 h correlate more closely with the long-term outcome two years and eight years later. [289, 415] It would seem much more useful to record the Sarnat grade at 48 h in every term baby suspected of intrapartum 'asphyxia' than to record the Apgar score. Early neonatal seizures are not always due to intrapartum stress: neither is early neonatal encephalopathy, but intrapartum stress is certainly the commonest cause of early encephalopathy in the term baby, and the chance that the encephalopathy is related to intrapartum events is enhanced if there is other evidence of organ dysfunction.

The threshold for recognising mild (Sarnat Grade 1) encephalopathy probably varies in different centres, but most units can expect to encounter 2–3 babies with Grade 2 or Grade 3 encephalopathy per 1,000 livebirths. Signs of encephalopathy need to be documented daily; better documentation of the duration of symptoms is likely to improve the prognostic power of the Sarnat grading system.

Summary learning

- **There is still much to learn about the optimum way to assist newborn babies make the transition to breathing air.**

- **Approaches, drugs and equipment that have been commonly used are being scrutinised to provide an evidence-based approach.**

- **Not all evidence will come from randomised controlled trials.**

My key take-home messages from this chapter

Practical procedures

Learning outcomes

To enable you to understand the indications for, the theory behind and the complications of the following procedures that may be encountered during newborn resuscitation:

- **Nasopharyngeal airway insertion**
- **Oral tracheal intubation**
- **Emergency needle thoracocentesis for management of tension pneumothorax**
- **Laryngeal mask airway (LMA) insertion**
- **Umbilical venous access**
- **Intraosseous (IO) needle insertion**

Introduction

The practical procedures covered in this appendix are technically challenging and, being practical skills, cannot be adequately taught in a manual. The indications, techniques and common complications of some of the more regularly performed practical procedures in newborn resuscitation and in neonatal intensive care are discussed here however the procedures themselves are best taught under direct supervision in controlled settings until competence is achieved. Only umbilical venous access is formally taught on the NLS course.

Nasopharyngeal airway (NPA)

Insertion of a nasopharyngeal airway (NPA) is designed to open the channel between the nostril and the nasopharynx. As most newborns are obligate nasal breathers this technique is particularly effective in this age group. An NPA is better tolerated by a conscious baby than an oropharyngeal airway. The technique is most commonly used to support a baby who has partial upper airway obstruction with patent nasal passageways and an adequate respiratory drive. This includes babies with congenital anomalies such as micrognathia, a large tongue (macroglossia) or other pathology causing restriction of the naso- or oropharyngeal spaces. [416-418]

The nasopharyngeal airway is a soft flexible plastic or silicone bevelled tube. Once sited the additional flange material may be cut down and used to secure the device in the correct position. Whilst there are specifically manufactured tubes for this purpose, a standard tracheal tube is, perhaps, more readily available in a labour ward and can also be used as a neonatal nasopharyngeal airway (Figure A2.1).

A correctly placed NPA will lie just above the epiglottis and separates the soft palate and back of the tongue from the posterior wall of the oro-pharynx. If the airway is too short it will fail to achieve this separation and if too long it can pass into the larynx and aggravate cough and gag reflexes. It is possible to estimate the length of the NPA required from the overall length of the baby [419, 420] but in the emergency situation, the length can be more readily estimated by measuring the distance from the tip of the nose to the tragus of the ear. Irrespective of the method chosen, there should be a significant improvement in the patient's respiratory status if the NPA is correctly placed and this too should guide the final length.

NLS

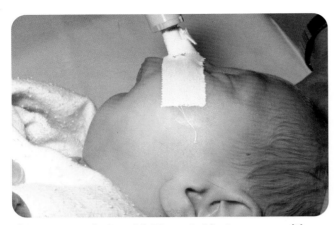

Figure A2.1 A baby with Pierre Robin Sequence with a shortened tracheal tube being used as a nasopharyngeal airway

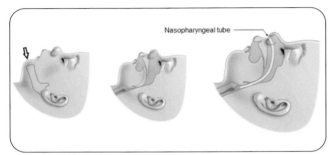

Figure A2.2 How the airway is obstructed in Pierre Robin Sequence and how a nasopharyngeal tube overcomes that obstruction

The size of the tube (diameter) can be estimated by visually matching its diameter against the internal diameter of the anterior nostril, although this is not always the narrowest part of the nasal airway and a smaller tube may be required if resistance is felt. [421]

The nasopharyngeal airway should be lubricated and introduced into the nostril with a gentle rotating motion passing the airway directly backwards and posteriorly along the floor of the nose. The length of the airway should be confirmed, if possible, by direct vision with a laryngoscope, observing that the tip of the device appears in view at the top of the oropharynx. The correct sized tube should fit snugly in the nostril without causing blanching of the nares.

This device is not suitable for infants with obstruction to the choanal space, significant coagulopathy or if there are copious or tenacious secretions.

Inserting a laryngeal mask airway (LMA)

The skills needed to successfully insert any LMA can be taught using neonatal manikin; after viewing a 15 min educational session using a manikin most people can insert an LMA in 15 s or less (mean time to insertion is five seconds). [422]

- Select the correct size. A size 1 LMA is appropriate for most newborn infants; the smallest baby that an LMA

can be used in weighs 1500 g.

- If the LMA has a cuff check that it inflates and deflates correctly (Figure A2.3a & b).

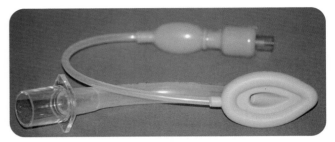

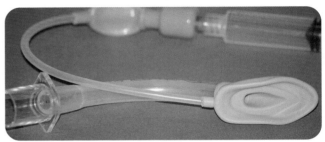

Figure A2.3a & b Inflate the cuff with the specified volume of air (a) and then deflate it again (b)

- Lubricate the LMA with water soluble gel.

- The LMA is held so that the opening is in a forward facing position (i.e. towards the baby's feet).

- The LMA is held 'like a pen' in the operators dominant hand with the index finger placed just above the cuff. The device is inserted with the cuff deflated (Figure A2.3c).

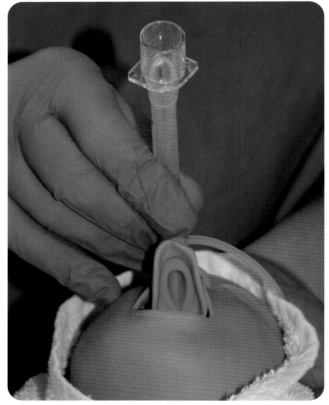

Figure A2.3c Inserting the LMA with the cuff deflated

- Position the head in a slightly extended position and introduce the LMA into the mouth. Slide the LMA downwards and backwards along the hard palate, to reach a resting position beyond the base of the tongue. A slight resistance to any further advancement will be felt (Figure A2.3d).

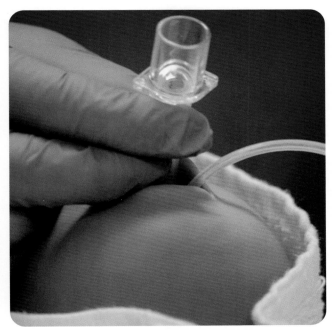

Figure A2.3d The LMA will meet with resistance once fully inserted

- Once positioned, the cuff, if present, should be inflated using an air filled syringe. A slight outward movement of the LMA will be observed when the cuff is inflated (Figure A2.3e).

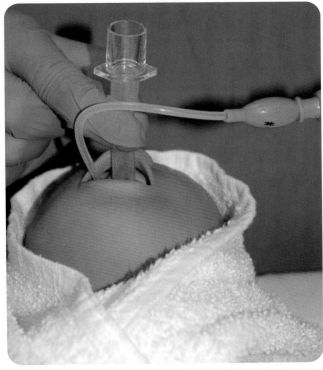

Figure A2.3e Reinflating the cuff of the LMA once it is in place

- A manual ventilation device attached to the LMA should achieve chest movement in the normal manner (Figure A2.3f).

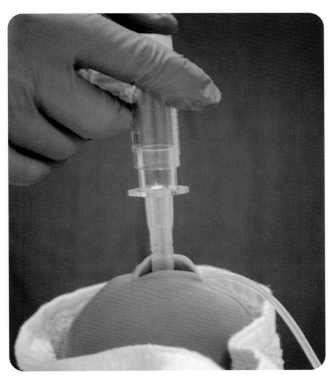

Figure A2.3f The T-piece being used to ventilate the baby

- The LMA should be secured in place using soft tape.

If the LMA has not been successfully inserted after 30 s the baby should be ventilated using a face mask before re-attempting LMA insertion.

The i-gel

The i-gel is a variant of the LMA that has a soft cuff that is not inflatable. [423] It may be available as an alternative (Figure A2.4a).

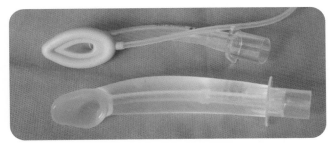

Figure A2.4a The standard LMA (top) and the i-gel. Both are supra-glottic airways; those pictured are size 1 airways suitable for neonatal use

The i-gel comes in a cage pack with the size clearly marked (Figure A2.4b). The i-gel is lubricated with a small amount of water-based lubricant taking care to ensure that there is no bolus of lubricant left in the bowl of the cuff. The technique for insertion is similar to that described for the LMA except there is no balloon to inflate.

The correctly inserted i-gel will protrude from the mouth slightly more than the comparable LMA due to the slightly longer overall dimensions.

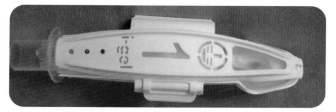

Figure A2.4b The i-gel in its cage pack with the size 1 clearly visible

Tracheal intubation

This manual can only discuss the practicalities of intubation. Tracheal intubation cannot be learnt from a book, a lecture or a video. Manikins currently available, even if they are 'intubatable', do not offer a sufficiently realistic experience and the best way is to be taught on an appropriately-sized anaesthetised patient by an experienced practitioner. Tracheal intubation can be performed by first passing the tracheal tube through the mouth (oral tracheal intubation) or the nose (nasal tracheal intubation). The latter, however, is technically slightly more difficult and tends to be used more in the elective setting.

Why intubate?

Most babies who are apnoeic at birth respond to lung aeration with a facemask [9] and intubation is unnecessary. It can occasionally be essential, for example, if the larynx or trachea is blocked with inhaled material. Intubation also provides a secure airway leaving the single-handed operator free to concentrate on other things and in preterm babies it allows you to give surfactant. Intubation, with the correct size tube, can also make the ventilation of abnormally stiff lungs easier. Surfactant deficient lungs, or 'dry' lungs following prolonged rupture of membranes (days or weeks) can sometimes be particularly difficult to aerate unless sustained pressures of 30 cm water or even higher are used at first. [126, 127, 424]

When emergency intubation is necessary it can be assumed that the baby is already limp, unresponsive and unconscious. Tracheal intubation in such circumstances is usually not difficult, although it is not a skill that staff should be expected to display without prior supervised experience. [267, 425-427]

> ## IT SHOULD BE POSSIBLE TO PLACE A TRACHEAL TUBE WITHIN 30 SECONDS
>
> ## IF YOU FAIL TO DO SO, REVERT TO MASK INFLATION BEFORE TRYING AGAIN

If a second person can check how long the procedure is taking and alert the operator if it is taking too long this can be helpful. [428] If tracheal intubation is proving difficult then managing the airway with facemask ventilation, possibly with a two-handed jaw thrust or oropharyngeal airway, ensuring good oxygenation and calling for additional help is important.

Tube size

Use the largest suitable tracheal tube – a snug fit is important. Too small a tube may not allow you to aerate the lungs especially if they are stiff or full of fluid (as at birth). If the tube is too small gas will escape through the gap between the tube and the tracheal wall and, if the lungs are at all stiff, so much gas will escape through the leak that they will not be inflated sufficiently. This can easily be detected by listening at the mouth or over the neck with a stethoscope while inflating the lung. Bubbles may appear at the mouth and chest movement will be poor. If you have chosen the right size tube and you can hear a large air leak you have intubated the oesophagus.

Tracheal tubes are classified by their internal diameter (ID) in millimetres. Tracheal tubes from different manufacturers may have different wall thicknesses and though it is the internal diameter that is most important from the respiratory point of view, it is the outside diameter that determines whether the tube will fit snugly into the larynx of any particular baby. For example 2.5 mm tubes can vary in external diameter from 3.5 to 4.1 mm and similar variations occur in other sizes. The size of tracheal tube can be estimated from the gestation at birth (Table A2.1). [429]

Gestation (weeks)	Birth weight (grams)	Size (mm)	Length (cm)	
			Oral	Nasal
25	650	2.5	6.0	7.0
28	1200	2.5	7.0	8.0
31	1600	2.5 / 3.0	7.5	8.5
34	2400	3.0	8.0	9.0
37	3000	3.0	9.0	10.5
40	3500	3.5	9.5	11.0

Table A2.1 A guide to tracheal tubes sizes and approximate lengths for oral and nasal intubation (Adapted from Kempley et al [429])

NLS

Tube length

If the tube is in the trachea, but has been pushed too far down and into one of the main bronchi (not always the right) then chest movement will not be symmetrical. A number of algorithms exist for judging tube length by weight, head circumference or foot length but a well-researched study has produced an algorithm based on gestation, which is the attribute most likely to be known at delivery (Table A2.1). [429]

Laryngoscopic intubation

Skilled emergency intubation depends on the prior acquisition of good technique. Develop a standard, planned and structured approach from the start. Many have found the following approach useful.

- Position all the equipment you need close by and prepare a means of securing the tracheal tube once it is in place.

- Position the baby on a firm flat working surface with the neck partially extended. A roll of blanket under the shoulders of the baby may help. (Do not over-extend the neck as this will stretch the trachea and position the larynx very anteriorly, making it more difficult to see and also making it difficult to push the laryngeal opening into full view using external pressure on the larynx).

- Position the laryngoscope. Hold the handle in your left hand while opening the baby's mouth. While looking down the laryngoscope insert it gently into the mouth. Be careful not to damage the gums.

- Position the tongue. In children and adults the usual approach is to insert the blade into the right hand side of the mouth and then to sweep the tongue into the left side of the baby's mouth by bringing the blade across into the centre during insertion. In newborn babies the tongue is usually relatively fixed in the floor of the mouth and it can be easier simply to slip the blade down centrally into the mouth over the tongue.

- Position the baby and yourself so you can see comfortably down the laryngoscope; if the surface the baby is on is height adjustable consider whether they are at the right height for you. If the blade is pushed in too far all you will see is the oesophagus (Figure A2.5a), you then have to withdraw the blade slightly to allow the larynx to drop into view from above (Figure A2.5b). Alternatively if the blade is not in far enough you may see little except the epiglottis (Figure A2.5c).

- Position the larynx. Once you have found the epiglottis, placing the tip of the blade at the base of the epiglottis where it meets the tongue (the glosso-epiglottic fold and the valleculae to either side) will bring the larynx into view from behind it (Figure A2.5d). Slight external downward pressure on the larynx may then help to bring the laryngeal opening into the centre of the field of view (Figure A2.5e).

- Position the tube. Bringing the tip in from the right hand corner of the mouth and keeping the curve of the tube horizontal so you don't obscure your view of the larynx (Figure A2.5f). A stylet is usually unnecessary if you have everything properly lined up but may be helpful if it is difficult to direct the tip of the tube into the laryngeal inlet. If the cords are tightly adducted wait for them to relax – don't prod. Reflex cord adduction proves that the baby cannot be in terminal apnoea. Insert the tube 1–2 cm through the cords and no further. The vocal cord guide marks, based on measurements in real babies [430], on the tube will help to judge this. However it is important to remember that the distance between the tip and the mark can vary according to the manufacturer and the internal diameter of the tube. [431]

- The airway is a tube, not a hole. Inserting a tracheal tube is passing one tube into another, not a tube through a hole. Try to ensure the tracheal tube is aligned with the airway otherwise it may be difficult to pass and may traumatise the fragile mucosa of the airway. This is especially important if using a stylet which makes the tube more rigid.

- Once the tube is passed gently remove the laryngoscope. The tube can be held in place against the hard palate by an index finger placed gently in the mouth.

- Aerate the lungs with five inflation breaths using a controlled inflation pressure of no more than 30 cm water (lower in preterm babies) sustained for two–three seconds, checking that the chest moves symmetrically. If available use capnography to confirm tube placement.

- Secure the tube immediately, while you know it is still optimally positioned and note the distance inserted by noting the markings at the lips. Be careful, it is easy to allow the tube to go down too far. If you do, you risk ventilating only one lung. Aerate the lungs with five inflation breaths using a controlled inflation pressure of no more than 30 cm water sustained for at least two seconds, checking that the chest moves symmetrically.

Confirming tube placement

The current gold standard for confirming tube tip position is a chest X-ray, however this is often delayed until after ventilation via the tube has been commenced. Rapid confirmation of correct tracheal tube placement at the point of care is important because tube malposition can be associated with serious adverse outcomes, including hypoxaemia, pneumothorax, lung collapse and death. After intubation, check that the tube is in the trachea:

- Check the heart rate – is it increasing? [432]

- Does the exhaled carbon dioxide detector confirm intubation? [356, 433]

- Listen at the mouth – is there a large leak?

- Look at the chest – are both sides moving equally? [434]

- Listen to both axillae – is air entry equal? [434]

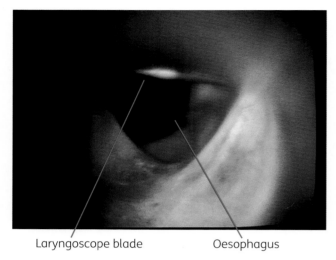

Laryngoscope blade   Oesophagus

Figure A2.5a The view seen when the laryngoscope is inserted too far

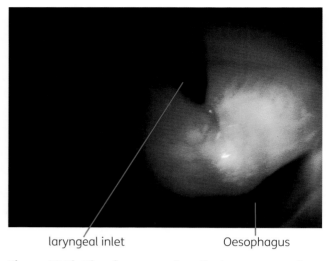

laryngeal inlet   Oesophagus

Figure A2.5b: The view seen when the laryngoscope is withdrawn slightly

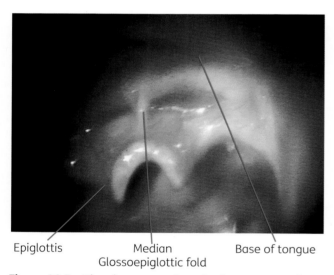

Epiglottis   Median   Base of tongue
        Glossoepiglottic fold

Figure A2.5c The view seen when the laryngoscope is not inserted far enough

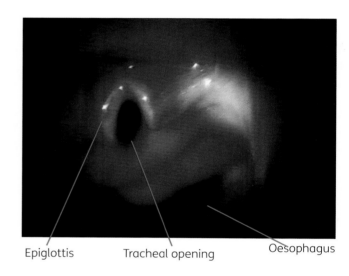

Epiglottis   Tracheal opening   Oesophagus

Figure A2.5d Inserting the laryngoscope in the glosso-epiglottic fold and vallecula to lift the epiglottis

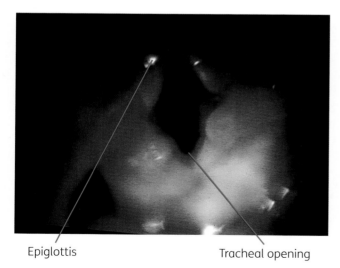

Epiglottis   Tracheal opening

Figure A2.5e Downward external (cricoid) pressure helping to bring the laryngeal opening into better view

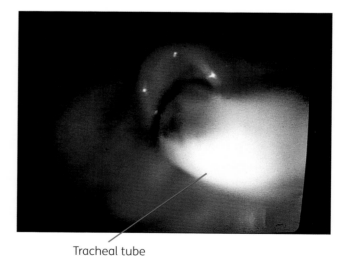

Tracheal tube

Figure A2.5f Inserting the tracheal tube

If the tube is in the right place, the chest will move symmetrically as pressure is applied, and the heart rate will usually start to improve within about 30 s. If the tube is not in the trachea there is likely to be a large leak around the tube which can usually be heard if you put your ear or a stethoscope to the baby's mouth while applying positive pressure to the tube.

Colorimetric CO_2 detectors

Studies suggest that detection of exhaled CO_2 confirms tracheal intubation in neonates with cardiac output more rapidly and accurately than clinical assessment alone. [435-437] Colorimetric CO_2 detectors are available for babies weighing more than 1000 g. However, it is possible to use them in smaller babies. [438] In babies weighing less than 750 g there may not be sufficient chest recoil, however, if the tracheal tube is thought to be in place, one or two chest compressions can provide sufficient volume of exhaled breath to register on the device.

Though capable of a very quick response, [439] there are limitations to the use of these devices:

- Liquids spilt on the detector, such as adrenaline, surfactant or gastric contents, can cause a colour change thus falsely suggesting that the tube is correctly placed. This may be detected as a constant colour change, whereas with a properly placed tracheal tube there may be variation in the colour during the respiratory cycle.

- One can be misled about a correctly placed tube if the cardiac output is so low as to fail to deliver sufficient CO_2 to the baby's lungs [439, 440]

- Intubation of the right main bronchus will produce a similarly positive result.

- Large airway leaks may decrease tidal volume delivered to the detector which can limit the accuracy of the CO_2 detector.

Using a colorimetric CO_2 detector:

1. Before starting, match the initial colour of the indicator to the colour labelled "check" around the detector window as shown in Figure A2.6a. If the colour of the indicator is different or darker than the area marked "check", do not use.

2. Intubate the patient.

3. Firmly attach the CO_2 detector to the tracheal tube; then attach the breathing device and ventilate the patient with six breaths of moderate tidal volume.

4. Compare the indicator colour in the window on full-end expiration to ranges printed on the detector cover. A correctly placed tube will result in a colour change. (Figure A2.6b).

5. If the results are not conclusive, it cannot be assumed that the tracheal tube is correctly placed. An intermediate colour change may occur in an oesophageal intubation due to retained CO_2 in the

oesophagus or in a correctly placed tube if the baby is already hypocarbic or if the circulation is at a standstill.

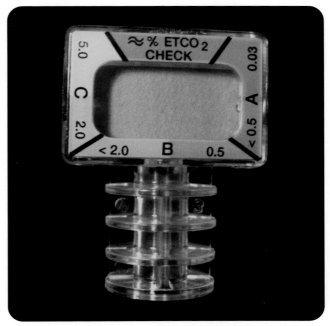

Figure A2.6a The unused CO_2 detector in which the colour matches the 'check' area

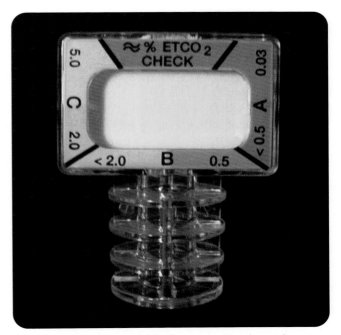

Figure A2.6b The used CO_2 detector showing colour change after exposure to CO_2

Teaching and practising intubation

There are many plastic models of babies designed for teaching and practising intubation but none provide an experience that is close to reality and some are frankly misleading. This important skill is one that is probably best learned by practicing real intubation in controlled circumstances under supervision from an anaesthetist in an operating theatre. Video laryngoscopes can be helpful when teaching intubation.

The ethics of gaining this experience by intubating babies after death has been extensively discussed amongst the medical profession but only a few have written of their discussion of this topic with the public. [426, 441] It is a practice that should perhaps not be rejected out of hand; provided the family, having been sensitively approached by a senior member of staff, agree to it.

In one study 32 of 44 families consented to this teaching being done with their dead baby, five families agreed to this but refused permission for autopsy, four families agreed to autopsy but not to intubation teaching. [426] Some families have later expressed satisfaction that their tragedy has been turned to some good in this way.

FACEMASK VENTILATION IS THE TECHNIQUE OF CHOICE IN NEWBORN RESUSCITATION

OTHER FORMS OF AIRWAY CONTROL MAY BE USEFUL IN SPECIFIC CIRCUMSTANCES

Emergency needle thoracocentesis

Needle aspiration (thoracocentesis) is the preferred immediate intervention in cases of tension pneumothorax where there is evidence of cardiorespiratory compromise. Signs of a pneumothorax include unequal chest movement, respiratory compromise and occasionally a displaced mediastinum. Pneumothorax can be confirmed using transillumination in small, usually preterm, babies but the thickness of the skin and thoracic walls, along with the lighting levels in a delivery suite, make this less effective in term infants.

There is usually insufficient time to obtain x-ray confirmation of a life-threatening tension pneumothorax, thus the diagnosis is a clinical one. There is, however, a 10–20% chance of causing a pneumothorax if thoracocentesis is attempted and the baby **does not** have a pneumothorax, thus the procedure should not be undertaken lightly.

- Clean the skin quickly using alcohol wipes. Allow the alcohol to dry before proceeding.

- Identify the site of insertion (this is the second intercostal space in the mid-clavicular line) by palpating the infant's sternum to find the manubriosternal angle (or angle of Louis). This marks the approximate level of the second pair of costal cartilages, which, in turn, attach to the second ribs. Follow the ribs along the side of the pneumothorax to the mid-point between both ends of the clavicle.

- Insert a 22G butterfly needle or cannula into the second intercostal space (i.e. below the second rib and aiming just above the third rib) perpendicular to the chest. Inserting the needle just above the third rib avoids the neurovascular bundles that run along the

lower borders of each of the ribs.

- As you insert the needle/cannula aspirate with a syringe until you get air entering the syringe. Do not drain the pneumothorax using this as the needle can damage the underlying lung.

- Alternatively, if you are using a butterfly needle the end of this can be held under water (e.g. larger ampoules of 0.9% sodium chloride or water for injection may be the most conveniently available). The entrapped air will bubble through confirming correct placement.

- Once stabilised consider insertion of a formal chest drain.

Umbilical vein catheterisation

Umbilical vein catheterisation is the most commonly used method for obtaining venous access in the newborn baby; intraosseus needles (see below) may be an alternative outside labour wards.

When to consider umbilical vein catheterisation

If the heart rate is still not improving despite good lung aeration, ventilation and a period of chest compression, then drugs or volume may be considered. Although umbilical vein catheterisation is seldom necessary in the emergency resuscitation of a baby at birth, it is a quick and effective way to gain access to the central circulation in a baby who has collapsed.

It can be critically important to be able to give volume replacement or drugs, to transfuse a baby, or to sample blood from a baby who is peripherally 'shut down'. Trying to cannulate a peripheral vein is more difficult, slower and will be totally ineffective for delivering drugs to the heart when the circulation is absent.

Equipment

Immediate access to a sterile pack containing all the essential equipment makes rapid and reliable umbilical catheterisation much easier. A basic pack could usefully contain:

- scalpel and a straight edged blade (e.g. No 11)
- 5 French gauge end-hole umbilical catheter
- three-way tap and 5 mL syringe
- two pairs of artery forceps
- one umbilical vein probe, some sterile gauze squares, a cord ligature or tape.

If this is a real emergency then there is no time for full aseptic technique, however you and an assistant should wear sterile gloves and observe universal precautions for your own safety.

Technique

Prepare the equipment. Fill a 5mL syringe with 0.9% sodium chloride and flush through a three-way tap attached to the umbilical catheter. Turn the tap to occlude the catheter to prevent air being sucked into the circulation should the baby gasp. Before you take a blood sample you have to aspirate back all the flush solution and a further 2-3 mL of blood to ensure there is no contamination of the sample for testing.

- Tie the cord ligature or tape loosely around the base of the cord. If a second twist is added to the tie (Figure A2.7) then it will hold if it is necessary later to pull it tight. The arteries are unlikely to bleed though bleeding from the vein is likely. However, arterial bleeding may follow recovery.

- Cut the cord 1–2 cm from the skin with a clean stroke of the scalpel. A sawing action causes 'teeth' at the vessel edge making catheterisation more difficult.

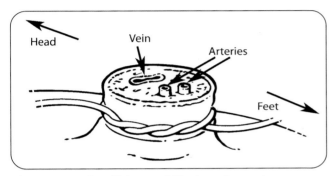

Figure A2.7 Identifying umbilical cord vessels

- Identify the umbilical vessels (Figure A2.7). There are usually two arteries and one vein; occasionally only a single artery is present. The vein travels 'north' (i.e. superiorly) from the umbilicus as the ductus venosus immediately beneath the anterior abdominal wall, passing through the liver to join the hepatic and portal veins then joining the inferior vena cava and entering the right atrium. The arteries are branches of the iliac vessels and enter the umbilicus from the 'south' (i.e. inferiorly). When the cord is cut close to the skin the thin-walled vein is usually found somewhere in the upper right quadrant, while the two stiff, string-like, white and bloodless contracted arteries are usually found somewhere in the two lower quadrants. Be sure to identify all three vessels.

- Grasp the cord with the artery forceps near the vein. With a second clip grip one wall of the vein before gently inserting the catheter into the vein using fingers or forceps. Do not probe the vein without supporting it by its edge with forceps. The umbilical vein may need to be gently dilated using a probe or a closed artery clip but is often easily entered without this.

- Advance the catheter until some resistance is felt at the umbilical ring just below the skin. Apply gentle pressure until the catheter passes through. The ideal place for the end of the catheter is within the inferior vena cava just outside the right atrium. In an emergency it is sufficient to get the end of the catheter in a large vessel – in other words into a vessel from which it is easy to aspirate blood.

- Draw back on the syringe and blood should flow back if the catheter is in the right place. If blood is not drawn back easily insert the catheter a little further or withdraw it slightly and try again. The first sample of blood can usefully be sent for pH, blood gases and haematocrit estimation.

- Flush the catheter gently with saline when in the right place to avoid thrombosis in the catheter.

- Secure the catheter. In an emergency, tape the catheter in place with one piece of tape across the abdomen. However, attaching adhesive tape to the thin skin of a preterm baby is best avoided because the catheter can easily be dislodged and on removal, the skin can be damaged. An alternative method for more permanent fixation is shown in Figure A2.8.

- Give drugs and 'fluid volume' if required.

Whenever possible umbilical catheterisation is best undertaken as a sterile procedure, in a properly equipped, warm, treatment area after the airway has been secured, and the circulation restored. It is also worth considering using a double-lumen umbilical catheter in such circumstances.

Securing an umbilical catheter

On the very rare occasions when this is needed as an emergency at delivery it almost always involves a term or near term baby. Under these circumstances the priority is to secure the UVC as central venous access. This can be done by taping the catheter securely to the abdomen.

If there is more time, one simple way to secure an umbilical catheter is to put two silk stitches into the substance of the umbilical cord, tie these in place and cut them about two inches long (Figure A2.8). Line these ends up alongside the catheter, turn the catheter back on itself and tape all together such that the catheter is taped to the silk. The catheter is then held securely in place with no tape attached to the skin. If it is necessary to adjust the catheter length after checking the position of the tip by X-ray or ultrasound this can be easily done.

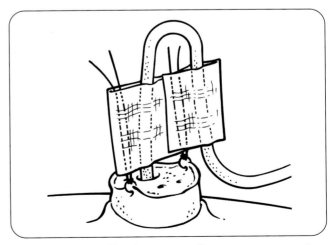

Figure A2.8 An effective system for more permanent fixation of umbilical catheters

Insertion of an intraosseous needle

Intraosseous needles have been used as emergency access in the event of failed peripheral, central and umbilical venous access in infants since 1943. [442] The technique was largely abandoned during the 1950s through 1980s with the introduction of plastic catheters that allowed more prolonged vascular access. [443] They are not commonly used in neonatal intensive care or in newborn resuscitation, but nonetheless can provide rapid central access through which both resuscitation drugs and emergency fluids can be administered. [222] In simulated newborn resuscitations they can be inserted as quickly as an umbilical venous catheter. [222, 223] The intraosseus route may also be useful in the very rare situation when a baby who has an abnormal looking umbilical cord and needs drugs. [224]

Technique

- There are different types of intraosseous needles; newer types are inserted using an automatic 'drill'

- Identify the insertion point on the anteromedial surface of the tibia, just below the tibial tuberosity

- Insert the needle applying downwards pressure until a 'give' is felt and the needle enters the bone marrow cavity

- Take any samples needed (notify the laboratory that they are bone marrow samples as the high white cell count in a bone marrow sample can be mistaken for leukaemia). Prioritise important samples such as glucose and cultures

Complications

Complications are rare but can be potentially serious: [444, 445]

- intraosseous needles should not be used if the bone is abnormal, (e.g. osteogenesis imperfecta)

- there is risk of fracture to the bone particularly in small babies [446]

- bone marrow embolism has been described.

> **DESPITE THE EASE OF INSERTION OF INTRAOSSEUS NEEDLES, UMBILICAL VENOUS ACCESS REMAINS THE EMERGENCY VASCULAR ACCESS PROCEDURE OF CHOICE ON DELIVERY SUITE**

Summary learning

- **The practical skills discussed in this appendix to secure an airway (nasopharyngeal airway insertion, tracheal intubation, laryngeal mask airway insertion), to drain a life-threatening tension pneumothorax or obtain vascular access (umbilical venous catheterisation, intraosseus needle insertion) are rarely needed in newborn resuscitation.**

- **These skills should only be undertaken by personnel who have been trained in these techniques and who are deemed competent to do so.**

My key take-home messages from this chapter

NLS

NEWBORN LIFE SUPPORT

Equipment – a discussion

Learning outcomes

To enable you to have a greater understanding of the following processes and pieces of equipment that may be encountered during newborn resuscitation:

- **Thermal care**
- **Working surface**
- **Facemasks**
- **T-pieces**
- **Self-inflating bags**
- **Pulse oximetry**
- **Stethoscopes**
- **ECG monitoring**
- **Suction**
- **Laryngoscopes**

Introduction

The basic principles which underwrite the approach to resuscitation at birth have evolved over the years through an incremental process and the same applies to the equipment used. The basic requirements are broadly very similar to those initially described in the 1960's during the phase when the approach we now take as standard was being developed.

More recently the approach to the management of the newborn baby has become less interventional, recognising the natural resilience of the newborn to cope with what are, otherwise, severe hypoxic insults and the need to 'first do no harm' (*primum non nocere*).

It is worth spending a little time reflecting on the equipment we use, and considering the finer points of application. Much will be discussed during the Newborn Life Support course, but time does not permit a detailed excursion. For those interested in this aspect, there is much to consider.

There is some value in reflecting on how the approach we adopt reflects the available technology. Large parts of the world lack the abundance of resources available in the National Health Service; how to deliver high quality resuscitation/stabilisation in such a resource-limited setting reminds us how much can be achieved with relatively little equipment – providing it is used intelligently.

Thermal care

For babies who are healthy the natural warmth of their mother is the best means of keeping warm as well as helping bonding. Delivering the baby onto the abdomen, then drying and wrapping it in such a way as to maintain skin-to-skin contact helps. Such an approach is equally valid for the late preterm baby who, following assessment is felt to be coping with breathing. Out of hospital, it is a valid means of supporting babies during their transfer to hospital at all gestations, providing airway and breathing can be maintained.

Should it be necessary to separate mother and baby for the purposes of assessment, stabilisation or resuscitation then consideration of the environment is vital. As previously discussed, modifying external factors such as using heaters, closing windows and minimising draughts is important. Within hospital, theatres are frequently adjusted for the comfort of the adults not the impending birth. It can be a challenge to get the temperature pushed high enough. The same may apply to any delivery area, whether this is in a hospital or not. It is important that you should be proactive on behalf of the baby.

Drying and wrapping is a tried and tested method of keeping babies warm that reduces convective and evaporative losses. It requires no more than the two towels, and whilst a radiant heater is helpful it may not be necessary for the mature, unstressed baby if the ambient temperature is appropriate. It is only when exposed that such adjuncts are needed or, in the case of the preterm, where undried, within the plastic bag an external heat source is obligatory to create the optimal environment.

Exothermic pads can be used in situations where a radiant source is not available and where kangaroo care is not possible but additional heat is required. [447, 448] They are useful in transfer situations and usually carried by transfer teams. Gloves filled with warm water can also suffice as an external heat source, but care needs to be taken not to scald the baby.

Working surface

In times past, the working surface of some resuscitaires had an angled front ostensibly to help keep the head in the neutral position. In reality, the presence of this slope led to over extension of the head, and a tendency for the baby to slip down towards the floor. What is required is a flat, non-slip surface that is firm, but cushioned, and insulated to prevent heat loss. Some platforms have offered active warming, but this is not required in general.

It is vital that the working surface is at a height that permits unhindered intervention. The floor may be the best surface in the community. In hospital, many resuscitaires have height adjustable platforms. A pre-requisite for effective intervention is to be able see what is going on. Having adequate lighting is important.

Recent developments have promoted delivery and assessment near the mother with delayed cord clamping. In recognition of this a number of devices have been developed which permit active management beside the mother, with bedside platforms (Figure A3.1) providing all the facilities of traditional resuscitaires. [449] Research is on-going to understand the implications and practice of intervention at the mother's side.

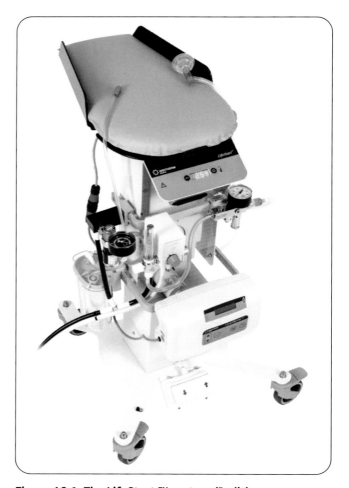

Figure A3.1 The LifeStart ™ system (Inditherm, Rotherham, UK) is one of a 'new' generation of resuscitaires that are designed to facilitate resuscitation and permit delayed cord clamping. Key features include adjustable height so that the baby can be placed in the right position for delayed cord clamping irrespective of type of delivery and that clinical staff can access the baby for resuscitation if required.

Facemasks

Facemasks are mentioned in Chapter 6. The function of the facemask is to permit gas under pressure to be delivered in sufficient volume to the lungs of the baby. The ability to achieve a good seal around the face is important. This attribute requires competent application. Even the best facemasks will fail in its function with poor use. [136, 144, 450]

There are two main types of mask (Figure A3.2); those that have a simple cushion of air which creates a seal through the application of downward pressure against the face, and those that have a thin cuff of deformable silicone where the pressure generated by the inflation breath pushes the collar against the face and makes the seal. Effective masks of this type typically have a very thick rigid upper section enabling even pressure to be applied downwards to make the seal. Both types of mask can be used to good effect if the correct techniques are applied.

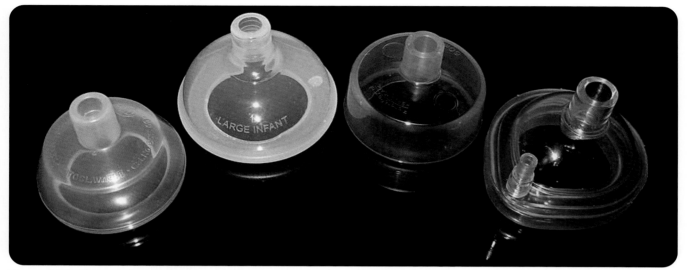

Figure A3.2 Commonly used facemasks for term babies from different manufacturers. From left to right; silicone round facemask (reusable), silicone round domed facemask (single-use), round silicone facemask (single-use), anatomical facemask with rigid upper section and inflatable rim (single-use).

It is vital masks are appropriately sized before use – it may be difficult to get a satisfactory seal on the smallest babies without a mask of appropriate size. When fitting a mask to a circuit make sure it is connected securely before applying to the face of the baby. It is not appropriate to try and reattach a mask whilst on the baby's face. Newer designs, such as the Laerdal mask on the right of Figure A3.2, have a flange to ensure the mask stays in place.

Be aware of the forces applied to the babies' face when mask ventilating. The pressure applied to ensure creation of a good seal is achieved through lifting the jaw into the mask as the mask is pushed down. Whilst for most babies these forces are not an issue, for the extreme preterm the force necessary to create a good seal may be significant, especially if the mask is a poor fit. [451] Be aware of the potential impact of mask support and avoid the tendency to simply push the mask down onto the face – without supporting the head/jaw sufficiently. The two-person technique is ideal in this respect.

T-pieces

The T-piece can only function if connected to a regulated positive pressure gas supply. Systems permit regulation of the flow of gas through the T-piece, the concentration of oxygen via a blender, and the pressure delivered. Most, but not all, T-pieces allow variation in the peak inspiratory pressure (PIP) and the level of positive end expiratory pressure (PEEP) through adjustable relief valves on the system, or the T-piece itself. Most systems have a secondary safety blow off valve – this is usually set to somewhere between 30 and 40 cm water. It is important to remember to adjust this if higher pressures are required.

When setting up a T-piece circuit it is important to check the level of PEEP and PIP before use. Some circuits are supplied with the PEEP valve screwed shut in which case potentially dangerous levels of pressure may be delivered

to the baby if used unchecked. The pressures delivered are flow rate dependent. Flows of 5–8 L min^{-1} are typical of those required. If the flow rate is changed, then the delivered PEEP will also change. [452, 453]

Flow is also important in determining tidal volume when the lungs are inflated. Whilst pressure is used as a proxy for tidal volume in the inflation and ventilation of babies, it is not the only factor to take into consideration. Although the pressure is an important factor it is the driving force that determines the delivery of a given volume; and the flow rate coupled to the inspiratory time is what defines that.

Bearing in mind the normal range of tidal volumes in a baby is only 5–7 mL kg^{-1} then once recruitment has occurred and the resting volume achieved, care needs to be taken. A 0.5 s inspiratory breath when using a T-piece (and when there is minimal leak) at 6 L min^{-1} will deliver 50 mL per breath. This is higher than the 17–25 mL tidal volumes in the average sized term baby, and certainly much higher than the tidal volumes of a preterm baby.

It is vital that the T-piece system is connected to a regulated supply, not direct to 'wall' oxygen which could result in dangerously high pressures and gas volumes being delivered. This is unlikely to happen if there is a means of blending air and oxygen in the system.

The advantages of the T-piece are that it is a simpler device to apply to the face of the baby than a self-inflating bag/valve system, especially for the single-handed resuscitator. [139, 454, 455] It has the ability to deliver adjustable PEEP through the screw valve on the circuit (Figure A3.3). In use, the T-piece delivers a more constant peak pressure for an operator-determined time interval. [456, 457] However, it does require a gas supply and thus cannot be used in situations where this is unavailable.

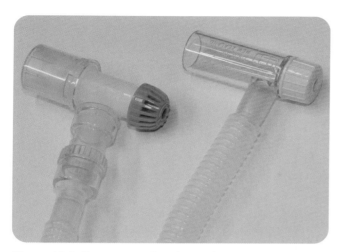

Figure A3.3 Two types of T-piece with adjustable screw-type PEEP valves.

T-pieces may be device specific or generic. Care needs to be taken as there are different fittings to enable connection to the gas supply. Some use the generic 15 mm connector; others have bespoke, narrower fittings requiring an adapter.

Self-inflating bags

Self-inflating bags provide gas under pressure in the absence of an external, pressurised supply. They are, therefore, useful in situations when such a gas supply is not available, in which case the inspired gas will be air. They can be used with an oxygen supply, allowing the inspired gas mixture to approach oxygen concentrations up to 90% if a rebreathe bag is connected.

The appropriate tidal volume during resuscitation is not known, most studies concentrate on establishing an adequate functional residual capacity (FRC) [61] and so we have to extrapolate from experience with spontaneously breathing babies at birth, ventilated babies after birth, and animal studies. For ventilated babies, with aerated lungs, a tidal volume of 4–6 mL kg^{-1}, at a rate of 40–60, provides adequate control of the partial pressure of CO_2. [458]

During the first inflations, where the fluid is moved out of the airways and an FRC is being developed, tidal volumes may need to be larger. Studies of colorimetric exhaled CO_2 detection and respiratory function, have shown that CO_2 may not be detected if the tidal volume is <3.2 mL kg^{-1}. [459] The tidal volumes for spontaneously breathing newborn preterm infants, however, ranged from 4.2 to 5.8 mL kg^{-1}. [460]

Despite our lack of knowledge of the appropriate tidal volume for the term newborn infant it is certainly less than the 500 mL that is the recommended size bag for resuscitation at birth. The reason for not recommending a self-inflating bag of smaller volume (e.g. 240 mL) is that these will not have sufficient volume to allow for

recruitment during sustained, 2–3 s, inflation breaths. Once the lungs are inflated, however, smaller volumes are required for tidal ventilation and smaller bags may be appropriate here. Using a larger self-inflating bag (i.e. 500 mL) in a less 'aggressive' way may provide these gentler ventilation breaths just as easily as the smaller bag (i.e. 240 mL). [461]

There are many different types of self-inflating bags. Some are single-patient use only, others require sterilisation between patents. Those used for paediatric and neonatal purposes usually have a pressure-relief valve in the circuit. This should be tested before use by occluding the bag outlet and squeezing. Once the pressure in the bag exceeds the blow-off pressure, the valve should open and flow be heard. The blow-off valve is usually a spring mechanism set at a pressure between 30 and 40 cm water. In use, the valve provides an indication of pressure delivery, however it **will not prevent** excess pressure/volume being delivered to the baby if the bag is being squeezed vigorously – in this case the inertia of the valve is such that a higher pressure may inadvertently be given.

> ## ALWAYS TEST THE BLOW-OFF VALVE BEFORE USING A BAG

Seal the outlet to the baby and squeeze the bag (Figure A3.4). You should hear the blow-off valve working as the pressure rises, if you do not hear this, check the valve mechanism. The valve may be faulty [462] or, in rare cases, be missing altogether as someone may have assembled the self-inflating bag using the connector from an adult bag. [463]

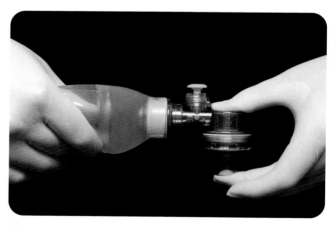

Figure A3.4 Testing the blow-off valve of the self-inflating bag

In use, the bag should be squeezed gently to achieve a pressure of about 30 cm water and sustained for 2–3 s. If the blow off valve is pre-set to 30 cm water, then activation of the valve will provide an indication that this pressure has been exceeded. Continued squeezing to just keep the valve open will allow delivery of a sustained inflation breath at the desired pressure. Aggressive squeezing will deliver higher pressures and excessive flow.

On rare occasions such as when faced with difficult to inflate stiff lungs in the mature baby pressures in excess of the blow off valve may be required. In such cases it may be necessary to override the blow off by preventing the valve operating through digital pressure. Care must be taken in these circumstances as unless there is some other means of monitoring the pressure there is no way to know the actual pressure being delivered.

Most self-inflating bags come with some form of oxygen reservoir (this can be a reservoir bag or additional tubing; and with re-useable devices this is also usually detachable). With air, this is a redundant device but when used with and oxygen supply this can allow the delivery of >90% oxygen because when the squeezed portion of the self-inflating bag re-inflates it draws oxygen from the source and from the reservoir. [161] If the reservoir bag is not used, but an oxygen supply remains connected, when the squeezed portion of the self-inflating bag re-inflates it will draw in air from the atmosphere and the system will deliver between 30-70% oxygen depending on the flow rate of oxygen. [159, 160] It is impossible to be precise about the amount of oxygen in these situations as there is no calibration.

The design of the self-inflating bag makes it cumbersome for the single person to use. The bag is at 90° to the direction of force required to make a good seal and the mechanics work against the operator in maintaining effective inflation. There are newer designs of self-inflating bag for neonatal use which have a simpler design with the bag oriented vertically, making it easier to hold and maintain an even pressure on the mask (Figure A3.5). These systems have been designed for use in health care systems where oxygen is not available and do not have a reservoir.

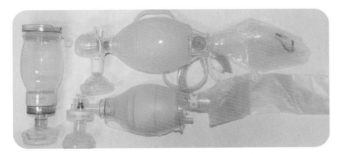

Figure A3.5 A selection of self-inflating bags. From left to right; a vertically-aligned, 'in line' self-inflating bag without reservoir – this has a smaller bladder and new design of mask with flange; (top) a single patient use 500 mL bag with fixed reservoir and valve with an override mechanism; and (bottom) a traditional self-inflating bag with removable reservoir.

Gas supply

Current evidence supports starting resuscitation of term infants using air. Supplemental oxygen is rarely needed. In the UK hospital setting all delivery areas will have piped, pressurised ('wall') oxygen and it is not unusual to have piped, pressurised air. Thus air/oxygen mixtures can be delivered by using blender devices, although parallel air and

oxygen flow meters can approximate the same function.

In the community, and in low resource settings, piped or cylinder gas is not usually available. If it is, it is usually oxygen, not air. Blended mixtures, therefore, are rarely used but a self-inflating bag may permit some variation in the delivered oxygen concentration as described above.

Flow rates of approximately 5 to 8 L min^{-1} are sufficient for the majority of interventions depending on the devices in use. The compliance of the baby's respiratory system will modify the rate at which the peak pressure is achieved. With non-invasive support, and significant soft-tissue dead space, the high compliance of the soft tissues buffers the low compliance of the lungs to slow the rate of pressure rise. When intubated this effect is removed, and the stiff lungs enable the peak pressure to be achieved very rapidly with potential risks. In this case, lower flow rates might suffice. If there are large leaks, either due to limited mask availability or endotracheal tube fit, then higher flow rates might be required to compensate.

Pulse oximetry

Pulse oximetry gives a quick and relatively accurate display, of both heart rate and oxygen saturation, easily seen by all involved in the resuscitation. This is particularly useful when stabilising significantly preterm babies or when tempted to give additional oxygen to any baby.

The pulse oximeter probe should be fitted preferentially to the right hand or wrist as this will give pre-ductal oxygen saturation values. However, fitting the probe takes time and the machine also needs to boot-up before it can start to give information. With practice, reliable data can be obtained within about 90 s of delivery. [464]

Set the data acquisition sensitivity to maximum and the data averaging time to the shortest available (~2 s). Once the oximeter is switched on, a reading can be obtained a few seconds faster if the probe is first attached to the baby and only then connected to the machine. [464] Once the pulse rate is displayed it is likely that this will be more accurate than other commonly used methods of assessing heart rate.

Be aware of the potential for artefactual readings – especially in situations of a poor cardiac output. Ensure a reliable signal is being processed.

Stethoscopes

Heart rate: Though it is often possible to assess the heart rate of a baby by feeling either for a pulse in the umbilical cord stump or by observing or feeling the pulsation of the ventricle against the chest wall, neither of these methods is reliable. [47] Detecting a heart rate accurately is much more reproducible with a stethoscope, even then it is prone to over-estimation. [465] If a stethoscope is used then it is important to get one with a chest-piece small enough to use on a small baby.

A stethoscope does not provide a reliable way of checking whether air is entering the lungs because the sound of air entering the stomach is all too easily transmitted into the chest. A stethoscope can, however, be useful in detecting cardiac displacement and in determining whether breath sounds are symmetrical between the sides of the chest.

Listening with a stethoscope at the mouth may help to determine whether a tube is in fact in the oesophagus. If there is a very audible leak when you apply positive pressure then it is likely to be in the oesophagus.

ECG monitoring

There is an increasing evidence base supporting the use of ECG monitoring as a means of rapidly determining the heart rate during resuscitation. [110, 111, 466] The ability to generate an ECG is determined by the ability to reliably place electrodes on the baby as well as by having necessary monitoring equipment in place at the right time.

Multi-parameter monitors capable of being used in the newborn setting are available, and the evidence suggests ECG monitoring can be used effectively. It has the advantage of giving an immediate indication of heart rate without delay providing the electrodes make effective skin contact. Ensuring effective contact can be problematic in the delivery room because of the newborn's wet skin and the possibility of skin stripping in premature infants, however these difficulties are not insurmountable. [110]

The ECG, however, indicates only the electrical rate of the heart – it provides no information on the effectiveness of any contractions. Just because there is an electrical heart rhythm does not mean cardiac compressions are unnecessary. Where there is dissociation between electrical activity and output, compressions will be required until output has been restored. This is the opposite of saturation monitoring, which depends on perfusion, and thus if there is a good pulse there is perfusion. Oximetry may give no indication of heart rate when there is cardiac contraction insufficient to generate a pulse.

Newer devices are being developed to enable the rapid determination of heart rate through ECG even in a low resource setting. This is perceived as more reliable than the stethoscope in untrained hands. These devices are designed to be robust, easy to apply and maintain with no disposable parts such as "stick on" electrodes.

Suction

The ability to clear an obstructed airway is essential whether it is in a hospital setting with wall suction, or in the community where portable devices need to be used. Whichever systems are used it is vital that the suction catheter is of sufficient calibre to enable removal of thick particulate material, which is more likely to cause a problem than thin watery secretions.
It is recommended that suction take place under direct vision in order to prevent inadvertent trauma to the

airway or stimulation of the pharynx leading to gagging and/or vagus nerve-induced bradycardia.

There are two types of suction catheter; rigid 'Yankauer' catheters, and longer, flexible catheters (Figure A3.6). Any catheter narrower than 12 French gauge is unlikely to be effective during resuscitation. Yankauer catheters have the potential advantage of a wider orifice, and can be directed with more precision but are rigid and thus need to be used with care. Their shorter length and tapered design means they are better able to cope with thick material than the long polyurethane catheters which will rapidly block as the length of tubing the material has to pass up is so long that is it difficult to achieve clearance. These catheters are fine for more liquid material. Where the trachea requires direct suction, then the ETT may suffice with a meconium aspirator (Chapter 6).

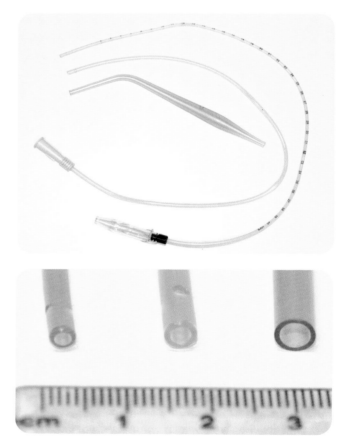

Figure A3.6 Three different types of suction catheter. The upper picture shows a flexible 10 FG catheter with control fitting (uppermost); a flexible 12 FG catheter without control fitting (middle) and a rigid Yankauer sucker, 15 FG paediatric type (bottom). The longer catheters will be much more likely to block with thick material than the short Yankauer. Note the difference in internal diameter as shown in the bottom picture, the Yankauer sucker (right) has a significantly greater internal diameter which combined with the shorter length makes it much more able to cope with thick particulate matter.

Laryngoscopes

Laryngoscopes are useful if there is a need to inspect the airway and, should the need arise, to permit visualisation of the cords and trachea for intubation. There are differing types of laryngoscope and blade. The shape of the airway makes a straight bladed laryngoscope appropriate for neonatal use. Adult laryngoscopes have curved blades.

As a rule, longer blades can be used in smaller patients, but the opposite is not true, so it is difficult to visualise the cords in a large baby with a very short blade. Blades are described by their name and size. There are a number of different types of blade and it is a matter of individual preference as to which is felt to be the best. Much of the time there is no choice: you have to use what is available. If there is a choice then being able to recognise the different attributes can be helpful.

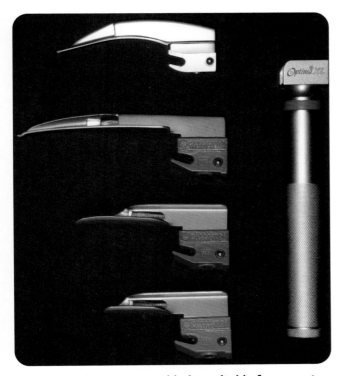

Figure A3.7 Laryngoscope blades suitable for neonates and small infants. The photograph shows (from top to bottom), a curved Macintosh paediatric blade (size 1), a straight Seward blade (size 1), a straight Miller blade (size 0) and a straight Miller blade (size 00). These are all fibre-optic blades with the handle containing the light source.

A variety of different types of laryngoscope blades are available and which are suitable for neonatal resuscitation. Typically a size 1 blade is used for larger babies, a size 0 blade for smaller ones and for the smallest babies a size 00 blade might be required (Figure A3.7). The Seward and Miller blades are among the more commonly available and typified by a flat blade with a smaller, non-curving, tongue-guard holding the tongue to the side. Wisconsin and Robertshaw blades (not shown) are similar. The Oxford blade (also not shown) is characterised by a very large tongue guard curving over to create a tunnel through which it is possible to see the airway. This can be a challenge to insert in very small oral cavities but has the effect of holding the structures open.

Most new laryngoscopes have a high intensity LED light source in the handle and a fibreoptic light guide in the blade. Blades may be re-useable or disposable. The quality of the light guide in the disposable blades, however, tends to be less effective, reflecting their cheaper construction.

Although unlikely to be routinely used in the newborn setting, there are also video laryngoscopes where the fibreoptic image from the blade is transmitted through to a video display. These can be useful in situations anticipating the 'difficult airway' and for teaching purposes.

My key take-home messages from this chapter

Antenatally diagnosed conditions that require forward planning

Learning outcomes

To enable you to understand which antenatal diagnoses might affect the resuscitation process and how to approach these infants if they are born unexpectedly:

- **Congenital heart disease**
- **Intrathoracic masses**
- **Conditions that might compromise the airway**
- **Neural tube defects**
- **Abdominal wall defects**
- **Skeletal dysplasias**
- **Renal anomalies**

In most cases, antenatal diagnosis allows for forward planning for the delivery of babies with congenital anomalies that are likely to require additional attention in the newborn period. This might include antenatal transfer to an appropriate centre, induction of labour or elective operative delivery so that optimum care can be given.

As with all plans, nature (and the baby) may have other ideas and the delivery may occur before the team can arrive or before the mother can be transferred to the tertiary centre. This section gives a brief overview of some of the more common anomalies (all of which are rare in themselves) and suggests how a person with basic newborn resuscitation knowledge and skills can support that baby until additional help arrives.

Congenital heart disease

Most cases of congenital heart disease do not, in the absence of hydrops, require additional support during the initial transition to extra-uterine life – even those with complex, ductal-dependent congenital heart anomalies. Those in need of resuscitation should be approached in the same way as any other newborn infant. Call for senior support as soon as possible. On-going management of the congenital heart disease can take place once the baby is stabilised.

Intrathoracic masses

This category includes congenital diaphragmatic hernia (CDH) and intrapulmonary lesions such as congenital cystic adenomatoid malformation (CCAM) or congenital pulmonary airway malformation (CPAM) and bronchopulmonary sequestrations, which may cause respiratory compromise in the newly born infant. The birth of any such babies would be planned in such a way that an experienced resuscitation team is available.

Many CCAM or CPAM reduce in size as the fetus approaches term and may be undetectable on ultrasound by the time of delivery. [467] These babies are unlikely to present with any significant respiratory problems and a standard approach to resuscitation should be followed if required.

Conditions that carry a high risk for neonatal airway obstruction

Airway obstruction may occur at any level of the airway, and may be caused by external compression or intrinsic structural abnormalities. The fetus with severe micrognathia may be at significant risk of airway obstruction at delivery. As before, the birth of any such babies would be planned in such a way that an experienced resuscitation team is available.

Babies with micrognathia may be manageable using some of the airway techniques described in this manual (e.g. two handed jaw support, oro- or naso-pharyngeal airways, etc.) and these procedures should be attempted before resorting to more invasive measures.

Neural tube defects (including encephalocoele and myelomeningocele)

The breathing of babies with encephalocoeles may be impaired because of airway obstruction or central apnoea. They usually require no more than routine resuscitation measures to correct this until such time that senior help arrives.

Babies with myelomeningocele generally do not have respiratory problems, however an associated hydrocephalus may cause the neck to be flexed and the airway to be compromised when in the supine position. In addition, steps should be taken to protect the exposed neural elements and prevent rupture of the membrane covering the defect; place the baby in a prone or side-lying position and cover the lesion with sterile saline-soaked gauze and a plastic wrap covering.

Abdominal wall defects (omphalocele and gastroschisis)

Thermoregulation and fluid loss is a concern here because the baby may lose heat through the exposed viscera, in addition insensible fluid loss is significant. A sterile plastic bag is often placed over the lower extremities and trunk to the level of the nipple line but another option to maintain bowel integrity is to apply warm, sterile saline-soaked gauze loosely around the lower abdomen and defect, after which the whole thing is wrapped in plastic wrap to limit insensible losses.

If positive pressure ventilation is required to support ventilation consider passing a nasogastric tube to minimise intestinal distension and expedite elective tracheal intubation. If vascular access is required it may be necessary to consider the intraosseus route (Appendix 2) in an emergency as umbilical venous catheterisation may be difficult.

Skeletal dysplasias

Good antenatal communications between obstetric, genetics, neonatal providers and the parents is essential to allow the resuscitation team to understand the current status of the fetus and most likely diagnosis, and thus the prognosis. Special consideration may need to be given to the possibility of pulmonary hypoplasia (where a higher pressure may be required) or bone fragility (where gentle handling is required). Chest compressions, if required, should not be withheld for fear that they may cause rib fractures. [200]

Renal anomalies

Renal anomalies are among the most frequently detected problems on antenatal screening and, in the presence of normal liquor volumes, do not usually present with additional problems that require consideration during resuscitation. If the liquor volume is reduced or absent then the baby may have severe respiratory problems due to pulmonary hypoplasia (Potter's sequence); higher pressures may be required to inflate the lungs but the prognosis for such infants remains poor. [468]

References

1. Wyckoff MH, Perlman JM, Laptook AR. Use of volume expansion during delivery room resuscitation in near-term and term infants. *Pediatrics* 2005;**115**:950–5.

2. Adamsons K Jr, Behrman R, Dawes GS, *et al*. Resuscitation by positive pressure ventilation and Tris-hydroxymethyl-aminomethane in rhesus monkeys asphyxiated at birth. *J Pediatr* 1964;**65**:807–18.

3. Akerren Y, Furstenberg N. Gastrointestinal administration of oxygen in the treatment of asphyxia in the newborn. *J Obstet Gynaecol Br Emp* 1950;**57**:705–13.

4. Aladangady N, McHugh S, Aitchison TC, *et al*. Infants' blood volume in a controlled trial of placental transfusion at preterm delivery. *Pediatrics* 2006;**117**:93–8.

5. Morley CJ, Davis PG. Advances in neonatal resuscitation: supporting transition. *Arch Dis Child Fetal Neonatal Ed* 2008;**93**:F334–6.

6. Kroll L, Twohey L, Daubeney PE, *et al*. Risk factors at delivery and the need for skilled resuscitation. *Eur J Obstet Gynecol Reprod Biol* 1994;**55**:175–7.

7. Information & Statistics Division, Scottish Health Service. Hospital and Health Board Comparisons in Obstetrics 1988-90.1992; 57.

8. Singh J, Santosh S, Wyllie JP, *et al*. Effects of a course in neonatal resuscitation—evaluation of an educational intervention on the standard of neonatal resuscitation. *Resuscitation* 2006;**68**:385–9.

9. Palme-Kilander C. Methods of resuscitation in low-Apgar-score in newborn infants – a national survey. *Acta Paediatr* 1992;**81**:739–44.

10. Allwood AC, Madar RJ, Baumer JH, *et al*. Changes in resuscitation practice at birth. *Arch Dis Child Fetal Neonatal Ed* 2003;**88**:F375–9.

11. Macfarlane A, Mugford M. Birth counts; Statistics of pregnancy and childbirth. Chapter 12. HMSO, London, 2000. p327–35.

12. Palme C, Nyström B, Tunell R. An evaluation of the efficiency of facemasks in the resuscitation of newborn infants. *Lancet* 1985;**i**:207–10.

13. Perlman JM, Risser R. Cardiopulmonary resuscitation in the delivery room. Associated clinical events. *Arch Pediatr Adolesc Med* 1995;**149**:20–5.

14. Primhak RA, Herber SM, Whincup G, Milner RDG. Which deliveries require paediatricians in attendance? *Br Med J* 1984;**289**:16–18.

15. Bland RD. Lung liquid clearance before and after birth. *Semin Perinatol* 1988;**12**:124–33.

16. Lind J. Initiation of breathing in the newborn infant. *J Ir Med Assoc* 1962;**50**:88–93.

17. Wyllie J, Perlman JM, Kattwinkel J, *et al*; Neonatal Resuscitation Chapter Collaborators. Part 7: Neonatal resuscitation: 2015 International Consensus on Cardiopulmonary Resuscitation and Emergency Cardiovascular Care Science with Treatment Recommendations. *Resuscitation* 2015;**95**:e169–201.

18 Wyllie J, Bruinenberg J, Roehr CC, et al. European Resuscitation Council Guidelines for Resuscitation 2015: Section 7. Resuscitation and support of transition of babies at birth. *Resuscitation* 2015;**95**:249–63.

19. Moss AJ, Monset-Couchard M. Placental transfusion: early versus late clamping of the umbilical cord. *Pediatrics* 1967;**40**:109–26.

20. Yao AC, Lind J. Effect of gravity on placental transfusion. *Lancet* 1969;**ii**:505–8.

21. Walker D, Walker A, Wood C. Temperature of the human fetus. *J Obstet Gynaecol Br Commonw* 1969;**76**:503–11.

22. Currie AE. How cold can you get? A case of severe neonatal hypothermia. *J R Soc Med* 1994;**87**:293–4.

23. Dahm LS, James LS. Newborn temperature and calculated heat loss in the delivery room. *Pediatrics* 1972;**49**:504–13.

24. Stephenson JM, Du JN, Oliver TK. The effect of cooling on blood gas tensions in newborn infants. *J Pediatr* 1970;**76**:848–51.

25. Gandy GM, Adamsons K, Cunningham N, *et al*. Thermal environment and acid-base homeostasis in human infants during the first few hours of life. *J Clin Invest* 1964;**43**:751–8.

26. Gluck L, Kulovich MV, Eidelman AI, *et al*. Biochemical development of surface activity in mammalian lung. iv. Pulmonary lecithin synthesis in the human fetus and newborn and etiology of the respiratory distress syndrome. *Pediatr Res* 1972;**6**:81–99.

27. A Abd-El Hamid S, Badr-El Din MM, Dabous NI, *et al*. Effect of the use of a polyethylene wrap on the morbidity and mortality of very low birth weight infants in Alexandria University Children's Hospital. *J Egypt Public Health Assoc* 2012;**87**:104–8.

28. Macintosh M. (ed.). Project 27/28. An enquiry into quality of care and its effect on the survival of babies born at 27-28 weeks. Confidential Enquiry into Stillbirths and Deaths in Infancy. The Stationary Office, London, 2003.

29. Bateman DA, O'Bryan L, Nicholas SW, Heagarty MC. Outcome of unattended out-of-hospital births in Harlem. *Arch Pediatr Adolesc Med* 1994;**148**:147–52.

30. Bhoopalam PS, Watkinson M. Babies born before arrival at hospital. *Br J Obstet Gynaecol* 1991;**98**:57–64

31. Boo NY, Guat-Sim Cheah I; Malaysian National Neonatal Registry. Admission hypothermia among VLBW infants in Malaysian NICUs. *J Trop Pediatr* 2013;**59**:447–52.

32. Mullany LC, Katz J, Khatry SK, *et al*. Risk of mortality associated with neonatal hypothermia in southern Nepal. *Arch Pediatr Adolesc Med* 2010;**164**:650–6.

33. Mullany LC. Neonatal hypothermia in low-resource settings. *Semin Perinatol* 2010;**34**:426–33.

34. Johanson RB, Spencer SA, Rolfe P, *et al*. Effect of post-delivery care on neonatal body temperature. *Acta Paediatr* 1992;**81**:859–63.

35. Manani M, Jegatheesan P, DeSandre G, Song D, Showalter L, Govindaswami B. Elimination of admission hypothermia in preterm very low-birth-weight infants by standardization of delivery room management. *Perm J* 2013 ;**17**:8-13.

36. World Health Organization: Department of Reproductive Health and Research (RHR) Thermal protection of the newborn: a practical guide (WHO/RHT/MSM/97.2) Geneva. 1997

37. Jia YS, Lin ZL, Lv H, *et al*. Effect of delivery room temperature on the admission temperature of premature infants: a randomized controlled trial. *J Perinatol* 2013;**33**:264–7.

38. Kent AL, Williams J. Increasing ambient operating theatre temperature and wrapping in polyethylene improves admission temperature in premature infants. *J Paediatr Child Health* 2008;**44**:325-31.

39. Fardig JA. A comparison of skin-to-skin contact and radiant heaters in promoting neonatal thermoregulation. *J Nurse Midwifery* 1980;**25**:19–28.

40. Bergman NJ, Linley LL, Fawcus SR. Randomized controlled trial of skin-to-skin contact from birth versus conventional incubator for physiological stabilization in 1200- to 2199-gram newborns. *Acta Paediatr* 2004;**93**:779–85.

41. Christensson K, Siles C, Moreno L, *et al*. Temperature, metabolic adaptation and crying in healthy full-term newborns cared for skin-to-skin or in a cot. *Acta Paediatr* 1992;**81**:488–93.

42. Christensson K. Fathers can effectively achieve heat conservation in healthy newborn infants. *Acta Paediatr* 1996;**85**:1354–60.

43. Bystrova K, Widstrom AM, Matthiesen AS, *et al*. Skin-to-skin contact may reduce negative consequences of "the stress of being born": a study on temperature in newborn infants, subjected to different ward routines in St. Petersburg. *Acta Paediatr* 2003;**92**:320–6.

44. Nimbalkar SM, Patel VK, Patel DV, Nimbalkar AS, Sethi A, Phatak A. Effect of early skin-to-skin contact following normal delivery on incidence of hypothermia in neonates more than 1800 g: randomized control trial. *J Perinatol* 2014;**34**:364–8.

45. Marin Gabriel MA, Llana Martin I, López Escobar A, Fernandez Villalba E, Romero Blanco I, Touza Pol P. Randomized controlled trial of early skin-to-skin contact: effects on the mother and the newborn. *Acta Paediatr* 2010;**99**:1630–4.

46. Chamberlain R, Chamberlain G, Howlett B, Claireaux A. Chapter 4. The first breath. In British Births 1970. Volume 1: The first week of life. Heinemann Medical, London; 1975. p.89–117.

47. Owen CJ, Wyllie JP. Determination of heart rate in babies at birth. *Resuscitation* 2004;**60**:213–7.

48. Nimbalkar SM, Patel VK, Patel DV, *et al*. Effect of early skin-to-skin contact following normal delivery on incidence of hypothermia in neonates more than 1800 g: randomized control trial. *J Perinatol* 2014;**34**:364–8.

49. Pejovic NJ, Herlenius E. Unexpected collapse of healthy newborn infants: risk factors, supervision and hypothermia treatment. *Acta Paediatr* 2013;**102**:680–8.

50. Becher JC, Bhushan SS, Lyon AJ. Unexpected collapse in apparently healthy newborns—a prospective national study of a missing cohort of neonatal deaths and near-death events. *Arch Dis Child Fetal Neonatal Ed* 2012;**97**:F30–4.

51. Fleming PJ. Unexpected collapse of apparently healthy newborn infants: the benefits and potential risks of skin-to-skin contact. *Arch Dis Child Fetal Neonatal Ed* 2012;**97**:F2–3.

52. Hoseth E, Joergensen A, Ebbesen F, Moeller M. Blood glucose levels in a population of healthy, breast fed, term infants of appropriate size for gestational age. *Arch Dis Child Fetal Neonatal Ed* 2000;**83**:F117–19.

53. Hawdon JM, Ward Platt MP, Aynsley-Green A. Patterns of metabolic adaptation for preterm and term infants in the first neonatal week. *Arch Dis Child* 1992;**67**:357–65.

54. Hawdon JM, Aynsley-Green A, Alberti KGMM, Ward Platt MP. The role of pancreatic insulin secretion in neonatal glucoregulation. 1. Healthy term and preterm infants. *Arch Dis Child* 1993;**68**:274–9.

55. Landon MB, Gabbe SG, Piana R, et al. Neonatal morbidity in pregnancy complicated by diabetes mellitus: predictive value of maternal glycemic profiles. *Am J Obstet Gynecol* 1987;**156**:1089–95.

56. Pruyn SC, Phelan JP, Buchanan GC. Long-term propranolol therapy in pregnancy: maternal and fetal outcome. *Am J Obstet Gynecol* 1979;**135**:485–9.

57. Hooper SB, Te Pas AB, Lewis RA, et al. Establishing functional residual capacity at birth. *NeoReviews* 2010;**11**: e474–83.

58. Te Pas AB, Davis PG, Hooper SB, et al. From liquid to air: breathing after birth. *J Pediatr* 2008;**152**:607–11.

59. Hooper SB, Harding R. Fetal lung liquid: a major determinant of the growth and functional development of the fetal lung. *Clin Exp Pharmacol Physiol* 1995;**22**:235–47.

60. Harding R, Hooper SB. Regulation of lung expansion and lung growth before birth. *J Appl Physiol (1985)* 1996;**81**:209–24.

61. Hooper SB, Siew ML, Kitchen MJ, et al. Establishing functional residual capacity in the non-breathing infant. *Semin Fetal Neonatal Med* 2013;**18**:336–43.

62. Gao Y, Raj JU. Regulation of the pulmonary circulation in the fetus and newborn. *Physiol Rev* 2010;**90**:1291–335.

63. Teitel DF, Iwamoto HS, Rudolph AM. Changes in the pulmonary circulation during birth-related events. *Pediatr Res* 1990;**27**:372–8.

64. Sobotka KS, Hooper SB, Allison BJ, et al. An initial sustained inflation improves the respiratory and cardiovascular transition at birth in preterm lambs. *Pediatr Res* 2011;**70**:56–60.

65. Peebles DM, Edwards AD, Wyatt JS, et al. Changes in human fetal cerebral oxygenation and blood volume during delivery. *Am J Obstet Gynecol* 1992;**167**:1916–7.

66. Walters DW, Olver RE. The role of catecholamines in lung liquid absorption at birth. *Pediatr Res* 1978;**12**:239–42.

67. Strang LB. Fetal lung liquid: secretion and reabsorption. *Physiol Rev* 1991;**71**:991–1016.

68. Bhatt S, Alison BJ, Wallace EM, et al. Delaying cord clamping until ventilation onset improves cardiovascular function at birth in preterm lambs. *J Physiol* 2013;**591**:2113–26.

69. Crossley KJ, Allison BJ, Polglase GR, et al. Dynamic changes in the direction of blood flow through the ductus arteriosus at birth. *J Physiol* 2009;**587**:4695–704.

70. Dawson JA, Kamlin CO, Wong C, et al. Changes in heart rate in the first minutes after birth. *Arch Dis Child Fetal Neonatal Ed* 2010;**95**:F177–81.

71. Brady JP, James LS. Heart rate changes in the fetus and newborn infant during labor, delivery, and the immediate neonatal period. *Am J Obstet Gynecol* 1962;**84**:1–12.

72. Adamson SL, Richardson BS, Homan J. Initiation of pulmonary gas exchange by fetal sheep in utero. *J Appl Physiol (1985)* 1987;**62**:989–98.

73. Adamson SL, Kuipers IM, Olson DM. Umbilical cord occlusion stimulates breathing independent of blood gases and pH. *J Appl Physiol (1985)* 1991;**70**:1796–809.

74. Condorelli S, Scarpelli EM. Somatic-respiratory reflex and onset of regular breathing movements in the lamb fetus in utero. *Pediatr Res* 1975;**9**:879–84.

75. Gluckman PD, Gunn TR, Johnston BM. The effect of cooling on breathing and shivering in unanaesthetized fetal lambs in utero. *J Physiol* 1983;**343**:495–506.

76. Cooper EA, Smith H, Pask EA. On the efficiency of intragastric oxygen. *Anaesthesia* 1960;**15**: 211–28.

77. Coxon RV. The effect of intragastric oxygen on the oxygenation of arterial and portal blood in hypoxic animals. *Lancet* 1960;**i**:1315–7.

78. Barrie H, Cottom DG, Wilson BDR. Respiratory stimulants in the newborn. *Lancet* 1962;**ii**:742–6.

79. Daniel SS, Dawes GS, James LS, Ross BB. Analeptics and resuscitation of asphyxiated monkeys. *Br Med J* 1966;**ii**:562–3.

80. Godfrey S. Blood gases during asphyxia and resuscitation of fetal and newborn rabbits. *Respir Physiol* 1968;**4**:309–21.

81. Eve FC. Actuation of the inert diaphragm by a gravity method. *Lancet* 1932;**ii**:995–7.

82. Eve FC. Complacency in resuscitation of the drowned. *Br Med J* 1943;**i**:535–7.

83. Handley DB, Handley D. A rocker for asphyxia neonatorum. *Br Med J* 1951;**ii**:1282.

84. Hemingway A, Neil E. An experimental study of different methods of artificial respiration. *Br Med J* 1944;**i**:833–6.

85. Cross KW, Dawes GS, Hyman A, Mott JC. Hyperbaric oxygen and intermittent positive pressure ventilation in resuscitation of asphyxiated newborn rabbits. *Lancet* 1964;**ii**:560–2.

86. Hutchison J, Kerr M, Williams K, Hopkinson W. Hyperbaric oxygen in the resuscitation of the newborn. *Lancet* 1963;**ii**:1019–22.

87. Cordey R, Chiolero R, Miller J Jr. Resuscitation of neonates by hypothermia: report of 20 cases with acid-base determination on 10 cases and longterm development of 33 cases. *Resuscitation* 1973;**2**:169–87.

88. Westin B, Miller J, Nyberg R, Wedenberg E. Neonatal asphyxia pallida treated with hypoperfusion and transfusion of oxygenated blood. *Surgery* 1959;**45**:868–79.

89. Azzopardi D, Strohm B, Edwards AD, et al. Moderate hypothermia to treat perinatal asphyxial encephalopathy. *N Engl J Med* 2009;**361**:1349–58 .

90. Gluckman PD, Wyatt JS, Azzopardi D, et al. Selective head cooling with mild systemic hypothermia after neonatal encephalopathy: multicentre randomised trial. *Lancet* 2005;**365**:663–70.

91. Shankaran S, Laptook AR, Ehrenkranz RA, et al. Whole-body hypothermia for neonates with hypoxic-ischemic encephalopathy. *N Engl J Med* 2005;**353**:1574–84.

92. Edwards AD, Brocklehurst P, Gunn AJ, et al. Neurological outcomes at 18 months of age after moderate hypothermia for perinatal hypoxic ischaemic encephalopathy: synthesis and meta-analysis of trial data. *Brit Med J* 2010;**340**:363c.

93. Dawes G. Chapter 12. Birth Asphyxia, Resuscitation and Brain Damage. In: Foetal and neonatal physiology. Year Book Publisher, Chicago, 1968. p.141–59.

94. Cross KW. Resuscitation of the asphyxiated infant. *Brit Med Bull* 1966;**22**:73–8.

95. Godfrey S. Respiratory and cardiovascular changes during asphyxia and resuscitation of foetal newborn rabbits. *Q J Exp Physiol Cogn Med Sci* 1968;**53**:97–118.

96. van Vonderen JJ, Roest AA, Siew ML, et al. Measuring physiological changes during the transition to life after birth. *Neonatology* 2014;**105**:230–42.

97. Safar P, Escarraga LA, Elam JO. A comparison of the mouth-to-mouth and mouth-to-airway methods of artificial respiration with chest-pressure arm-lift methods. *N Engl J Med* 1958;**258**:671–7.

98. Kouwenhoven WB, Jude JR, Knickerbocker GG. Closed-chest cardiac massage. *JAMA* 1960;**173**:1064–7.

99. Moya F, James LS, Bernard E, Hanks EC. Closed chest cardiac massage in the newborn. *Anaesthesiol* 1961;**22**:644–5.

100. Hamer Hodges RJ, Tunstall ME, Knight RF, Wilson EJ. Endotracheal aspiration and oxygenation in resuscitation of the newborn. *Br J Anaesth* 1960;**32**:9–15.

101. Tunstall ME, Hodges RJH. A sterile disposable neonatal tracheal tube. *Lancet* 1961;**i**:146.

102. Flagg PJ. The treatment of asphyxia in the newborn. *JAMA* 1928;**91**:788–91.

103. Blaikley LB, Gibberd GF. Asphyxia neonatorum: its treatment by tracheal intubation. *Lancet* 1935;**i**:736–9.

104. Apgar V. A proposal for a new method of evaluation of the newborn infant. *Anesth Analg (Clev)* 1953;**32**:260–7.

105. Moore WMO, Davis JA. Response of the newborn rabbit to acute anoxia and variations due to narcotic agents. *Br J Anaesth* 1966;**38**:787–92.

106. Hey E, Kelly J. Gaseous exchange during endotracheal ventilation for asphyxia at birth. *J Obstet Gynaecol Br Commonw* 1968;**75**:414–23.

107. Ditchburn RK, Hull D, Segall MM. Oxygen uptake during and after positive-pressure ventilation for the resuscitation of asphyxiated newborn infants. *Lancet* 1966;**ii**:1096–9.

108. O'Donnell CPF, Kamlin COF, Davis PG, et al. Clinical assessment of infant colour at delivery. *Arch Dis Child Fetal Neonatal Ed* 2007;**92**:F465–7.

109. Smit M, Dawson JA, Ganzeboom A, et al. Pulse oximetry in newborns with delayed cord clamping and immediate skin-to-skin contact. *Arch Dis Child Fetal Neonatal Ed* 2014;**99**:F309–14.

110. Katheria A, Rich W, Finer N. Electrocardiogram provides a continuous heart rate faster than oximetry during neonatal resuscitation. *Pediatrics* 2012;**130**:e1177–81.

111. Mizumoto H, Tomotaki S, Shibata H, et al. Electrocardiogram shows reliable heart rates much earlier than pulse oximetry during neonatal resuscitation. *Pediatr Int* 2012;**54**:205–7.

112. Dawson JA, Kamlin CO, Vento M, et al. Defining the reference range for oxygen saturation for infants after birth. *Pediatrics* 2010;**125**:e1340–7.

113. Falciglia HS, Henderschott C, Potter P, Helmchen R. Does De Lee suction at the perineum prevent meconium aspiration syndrome. *Am J Obstet Gynecol* 1992;**167**:1243–9.

114. Chettri S, Adhisivam B, Bhat BV. Endotracheal suction for nonvigorous neonates born through meconium stained amniotic fluid: a randomized controlled trial. *J Pediatr* 2015;**166**:1208–13.e1.

115. Hull D. Lung expansion and ventilation during resuscitation of asphyxiated newborn infants. *J Pediatr* 1969;**75**:47–58.

116. Vyas H, Milner AD, Hopkin IE, Boon AW. Physiologic responses to prolonged and slow rise inflation in the resuscitation of the asphyxiated newborn infant. *J Pediatr* 1981;**99**:635–9.

117. Stenson B. Resuscitation of extremely preterm infants: The influence of positive pressure, surfactant replacement and supplemental oxygen on outcome. In Hansen TN, McIntosh N (eds). Current Topics in Neonatology. No 4. WB Saunders, London, 2000.

118. Schmölzer GM, Kamlin COF, Dawson JA, et al. Respiratory monitoring of neonatal resuscitation. *Arch Dis Child Fetal Neonatal Ed* 2010;**95**:F295–303.

119. te Pas AB, Walther FJ. A randomized, controlled trial of delivery-room respiratory management in very preterm infants. *Pediatrics* 2007;**120**:322–9.

120. Stephens RH, Benjamin AR, Walters DV. Volume and protein concentration of epithelial lining liquid in perfused in situ postnatal sheep lungs. *Am J Physiol* 1996;**80**:1911–20.

121. Hooper SB, Kitchen MJ, Siew ML, et al. Imaging lung aeration and lung liquid clearance at birth using phase contrast X-ray imaging. *Clin Exp Pharmacol Physiol* 2009;**36**:117–25.

122. Madar J, Richmond S, Hey E. Surfactant-deficient respiratory distress after elective delivery at 'term'. *Acta Paediatr* 1999;**88**:1244–8.

123. Milner AD, Saunders RA. Pressure and volume changes in the first breath of human neonates. *Arch Dis Child* 1977;**52**:918–24.

124. Siew ML, Wallace MJ, Kitchen MJ, et al. Inspiration regulates the rate and temporal pattern of lung liquid clearance and lung aeration at birth. *J Appl Physiol (1985)* 2009;**106**:1888–95.

125. Boon AW, Milner AD, Hopkin IE. Physiological responses of the newborn infant to resuscitation. *Arch Dis Child* 1979;**54**:492–8.

126. Upton CJ, Milner AD. Endotracheal resuscitation of neonates using a rebreathing bag. *Arch Dis Child* 1991;**66**:39–42.

127. Hey E, Hull D. Lung function at birth in babies developing respiratory distress. *J Obstet Gynaecol Br Commonw* 1971;**78**:1137–46.

128. Oddie S, Wyllie J, Scally A. Use of self-inflating bags for neonatal resuscitation. *Resuscitation* 2005;**67**:109–12.

129. Meltzer SJ. Simple devices for effective artificial respiration in emergencies. *JAMA* 1913;**60**:1407–10.

130. Henderson Y. The prevention and treatment of asphyxia in the newborn. *JAMA* 1928;**90**:583–6.

131. Johnson KG, Babson SG. Resuscitation of the apneic premature infant. *Pediatrics* 1967;**40**:99–100.

132. Hoskyns EW, Milner AD, Hopkins IE. A simple method of facemask resuscitation at birth. *Arch Dis Child* 1987;**62**:376–8.

133. Wood FE, Morley CJ. Face mask ventilation – the dos and don'ts. *Semin Fetal Neonatal Med* 2013;**18**:344–51.

134. Wood FE, Platten CR, Byrne S, Wyllie JP. Manikin based studies of simulated resuscitation practices: Term Face Mask Study. *Pediatr Res* 2011;**70**:752 (abstract).

135. Wood FE, Platten CR, Byrne S, Wyllie JP. Manikin based studies of simulated resuscitation practices: Preterm Face Mask Study. *Pediatr Res* 2011;**70**:104 (abstract).

136. Wood FE, Morley CJ, Dawson JA, et al. Assessing the effectiveness of two round neonatal resuscitation masks: study 1. *Arch Dis Child Fetal Neonatal Ed* 2008;**93**:F235–7.

137. Wood FE, Morley CJ, Dawson JA, et al. Improved techniques reduce face mask leak during simulated neonatal resuscitation: study 2. *Arch Dis Child Fetal Neonatal Ed* 2008;**93**:F230–4.

138. Finer NN, Rich W, Craft A, Henderson C. Comparison of methods of bag and mask ventilation for neonatal resuscitation. *Resuscitation* 2001;**49**:299–305.

139. Bennett S, Finer NN, Rich W, Vaucher Y. A comparison of three neonatal resuscitation devices. *Resuscitation* 2005;**67**:113–8.

140. Dawson JA, Schmolzer GM, Kamlin CO, et al. Oxygenation with T-piece versus self-inflating bag for ventilation of extremely preterm infants at birth: a randomized controlled trial. *J Pediatr* 2011;**158**:912–8e1-2.

141. Szyld E, Aguilar A, Musante GA, et al; Delivery Room Ventilation Devices Trial Group. Comparison of devices for newborn ventilation in the delivery room. *J Pediatr* 2014;**165**:234–9.e3.

142. Morley CJ, Dawson JA, Stewart MJ, et al. The effect of a PEEP valve on a Laerdal neonatal self-inflating resuscitation bag. *J Paediatr Child Health* 2010;**46**:51–6.

143. Nimbalkar SM, Rao Pn S, Nesargi SV, et al. Comparison of efficacy of three devices of manual positive pressure ventilation: a mannequin-based study. *Ital J Pediatr* 2015;**41**:25.

144. Tracy MB, Klimek J, Coughtrey H, et al. Mask leak in one-person mask ventilation compared to two-person in a newborn infant manikin study. *Arch Dis Child Fetal Neonatal Ed* 2011;**96**:F195–200.

145. Maskery S. Neonatal resuscitation. *Clin Risk* 2008;**14**:46–8.

146. Mead J. Paediatricians negligent in emergency: Antoniades v East Sussex Hospitals NHS Trust (High Court, 16/03/07 - Mackay J). *Clin Risk* 2008;**14**:82–3.

147. Plaat F. The team needs a leader. *Clin Risk* 2008;**14**:43–5.

148. Wiswell TE, Tuggle JM, Turner BS. Meconium aspiration syndrome: have we made a difference? *Pediatrics* 1990;**85**:715–21.

149. Dillard RG. Neonatal tracheal aspiration of meconium-stained infants. *J Pediatr* 1977;**90**:163–4.

150. Marshall R, Tyrala E, McAlister W, et al. Meconium aspiration syndrome: neonatal and follow-up study. *Am J Obstet Gynecol* 1978;**131**:672–6.

151. Davis RO, Philips JB, Harris BA, et al. Fatal meconium aspiration syndrome occurring despite airway management considered appropriate. *Am J Obstet Gynecol* 1985;**151**:731–6.

152. Dooley SL, Pesavento DJ, Depp R, et al. Meconium below the vocal cords at delivery: correlation with intrapartum events. *Am J Obstet Gynecol* 1985;**153**:767–70.

153. Stubblefield PG, Berek JS. Perinatal mortality in term and post-term births. *Obstet Gynecol* 1980;**56**:676–82.

154. Turbeville DF, McCaffree MA, Block MF, et al. In utero distal pulmonary meconium aspiration. *South Med J* 1979;**72**:535–6.

155. Nangia S, Sunder SS, Tiwari S, et al. Role of endotracheal suction on the occurrence of meconium aspiration syndrome (MAS) in nonvigorous meconium stained neonates - a randomized controlled trial. E-PAS 2014;4680.1.

156. Katz VL, Bowes WA Jr. Meconium aspiration syndrome: Reflections on a murky subject. *Am J Obstet Gynecol* 1992;**166**:171–83.

157. Vain NE, Szyld EG, Prudent LM, et al. Oropharyngeal and nasopharyngeal suctioning of meconium-stained neonates before delivery of their shoulders: multicentre, randomised controlled trial. *Lancet* 2004;**364**:597–602.

158. Wiswell TE, Gannon CM, Jacob J, et al. Delivery room management of the apparently vigorous meconium-stained neonate: results of the multicenter international collaborative trial. *Pediatrics* 2000;**105**:1–7.

159. Thió M, Bhatia R, Dawson JA, Davis PG. Oxygen delivery using neonatal self-inflating resuscitation bags without a reservoir. *Arch Dis Child Fetal Neonatal Ed* 2010;**95**:F315–9.

160. Reise K, Monkman S, Kirpalani H. The use of the Laerdal infant resuscitator results in the delivery of high oxygen fractions in the absence of a blender. *Resuscitation* 2009;**80**:120–5 .

161. Finer NN, Barrington KJ, Al-Fadley F, et al. Limitations of self-inflating resuscitators. *Pediatrics* 1986;**77**:417-20.

162. Schmölzer GM, Agarwal M, Kamlin CO, et al. Supraglottic airway devices during neonatal resuscitation: an historical perspective, systematic review and meta-analysis of available clinical trials. *Resuscitation* 2013;**84**:722–30.

163. Singh R. Controlled trial to evaluate the use of LMA for neonatal resuscitation. *J Anaesth Clin Pharmacol.* 2005;**21**:303–6.

164. Zhu XY, Lin BC, Zhang QS, et al. A prospective evaluation of the efficacy of the laryngeal mask airway during neonatal resuscitation. *Resuscitation* 2011;**82**:1405–9.

165. Feroze F, Masood N, Khuwaja A, et al. Neonatal Resuscitation: The use of Laryngeal Mask Airway. *Professional Med J* 2008;**15**:148–52.

166. Tonkin SL, Davis SL, Gunn TR. Nasal route for infant resuscitation by mothers. *Lancet* 1995;**345**:1353–4.

167. Finer NN, Horbar JD, Carpenter JH. Cardiopulmonary resuscitation in the very low birth weight infant: The Vermont Oxford network experience. *Pediatrics* 1999;**104**:428–34.

168. Wyckoff MH, Perlman JM. Letter to the Editor: cardiopulmonary resuscitation in very low birth weight infants. *Pediatrics* 2000;**106**:618–20.

169. Jankov RP, Asztalos EV, Skidmore MB. Favorable neurological outcomes following delivery room cardiopulmonary resuscitation of infants < or = 750 g at birth. *J Paediatr Child Health* 2000;**36**:19–22.

170. Hake TG. Studies on ether and chloroform from Professor Schiff's physiological laboratory. *Practitioner* 1874;**12**: 241.

171. Schiff M. Ueber direkte reizung der herzoberflaeche. *Arch Ges Physiol* 1882;**28**:200.

172. Boehm R. Ueber wiederbelebung nach vergiftungen und asphyxia. *Arch Exp Pathol Pharm* 1878;**8**:68.

173. Maass F. Die methode der wiederbelebung bei herztod nach chloroformeinathmung. *Berlin Klin Wochenschr* 1892;**29**:265–8.

174. Galos G, Surks S. Cardiorespiratory arrest in the newborn treated by cardiac massage. *Am J Obstet Gynecol* 1957;**74**:1108–11.

175. Reilly RJ, Melville HA. Cardiac massage in the resuscitation of a stillborn infant. *Br Med J* 1962;**i**:91–2.

176. Halperin M. Heart massage in a newborn infant. *JAMA* 1957;**164**:1996.

177. Sutherland JM, Epple HH. Cardiac massage of stillborn infants. *Obstet Gynecol* 1961;**18**:182–6.

178. Gallagher B, Neligan G. Resuscitation of the stillborn infant. *Br Med J* 1962;**i**:400.

179. Thaler MM, Stobie GHC. An improved technic of external cardiac compression in infants and young children. *N Engl J Med* 1963;**269**:606–10.

180. Rudikoff MT, Maughan WL, Effron M, et al. Mechanisms of blood flow during cardiopulmonary resuscitation. *Circulation* 1980;**61**:345–52.

181. Del Guercio LRM, Coomaraswamy RP, State D. Cardiac output and other hemodynamic variables during external cardiac massage in man. *N Engl J Med* 1963;**269**:1398–404.

182. Voorhees WD, Babbs CF, Tacker WA. Regional blood flow during cardiopulmonary resuscitation in dogs. *Crit Care Med* 1980;**8**:134–6.

183. Berg RA, Sanders AB, Kern KB, et al. Adverse effects of interrupting chest compressions for rescue breathing during cardiopulmonary resuscitation for ventricular fibrillation cardiac arrest. *Circulation* 2001;**104**:2465–70.

184. Todres ID, Rogers MC. Methods of external cardiac massage in the newborn infant. *J Pediatr* 1975;**86**:781–2.

185. Menegazzi JJ, Auble TE, Nicklas KA, Hosack GM, Rack L, Goode JS. Two-thumb versus two-finger chest compression during CPR in a swine infant model of cardiac arrest. *Ann Emerg Med* 1993;**22**:240–3.

186. Houri PK, Frank LR, Menegazzi JJ, Taylor R. A randomized, controlled trial of two-thumb vs two-finger chest compression in a swine infant model of cardiac arrest. *Prehosp Emerg Care* 1997;**1**:65–7.

187. Dorfsman ML, Menegazzi JJ, Wadas RJ, Auble TE. Two-thumb vs two-finger chest compression in an infant model of prolonged cardiopulmonary resuscitation. *Acad Emerg Med* 2000;**7**:1077–82.

188. David R. Closed chest cardiac massage in the newborn infant. *Pediatrics* 1988;**81**:552–4.

189. Whitelaw CC, Slywka B, Goldsmith LJ. Comparison of a two-finger versus two-thumb method for chest compressions by healthcare providers in an infant mechanical model. *Resuscitation* 2000;**43**:213–6.

190. Christman C, Hemway RJ, Wyckoff MH, Perlman JM. The two-thumb is superior to the two-finger method for administering chest compressions in a manikin model of neonatal resuscitation. *Arch Dis Child Fetal Neonatal Ed* 2011;**96**:F99–101.

191. Phillips GW, Zideman DA. Relation of the infant heart to sternum: its significance in cardiopulmonary resuscitation. *Lancet* 1986;**i**:1024–5.

192. Orlowski JP. Optimum position for external cardiac compression in infants and young children. *Ann Emerg Med* 1986;**5**:667–73.

193. Finholt DA, Kettick RG, Wagner HR, et al. The heart is under the lower one third of the sternum. *Am J Dis Child* 1986;**140**:646–9.

194. Clements F, McGowan J. Finger position for chest compressions in cardiac arrest in infants. *Resuscitation* 2000;**44**:43–6.

195. Lee SH, Cho YC, Ryu S, et al. A comparison of the area of chest compression by the superimposed-thumb and the alongside-thumb techniques for infant cardiopulmonary resuscitation. *Resuscitation* 2011;**82**:1214–7.

196. Lim JS, Cho Y, Ryu S, et al. Comparison of overlapping (OP) and adjacent thumb positions (AP) for cardiac compressions using the encircling method in infants. *Emerg Med J* 2013;**30**:139–42.

197. Meyer A, Nadkarni V, Pollock A, et al. Evaluation of the Neonatal Resuscitation Program's recommended chest compression depth using computerized tomography imaging. *Resuscitation* 2010;**81**:544–8.

198. Maher KO, Berg RA, Lindsey CW, et al. Depth of sternal compression and intra-arterial blood pressure during CPR in infants following cardiac surgery. *Resuscitation* 2009;**80**:662–4.

199. Spevak MR, Kleinman PK, Belanger PL, et al. Cardiopulmonary resuscitation and rib fractures in infants; a postmortem radiologic pathologic study. *JAMA* 1994;**272**:617–8.

200. Sewell RD, Steinberg MA. Chest compressions in an infant with osteogenesis imperfect type II: no new rib fractures. *Pediatrics* 2000;**106**:e71.

201. Dean JM, Koehler RC, Schleien CL, et al. Age-related effects of compression rate and duration in cardiopulmonary resuscitation. *J Appl Physiol* 1990;**68**:554–60.

202. Whyte SD, Sinha AK, Wyllie JP. Neonatal resuscitation – a practical assessment. *Resuscitation* 1999;**40**:21–5.

203. Li ES, Cheung PY, O'Reilly M, Aziz K, Schmölzer GM. Rescuer fatigue during simulated neonatal cardiopulmonary resuscitation. *J Perinatol* 2015;**35**:142–5.

204. Kern KB, Hilwig RW, Berg RA, et al. Importance of continuous chest compressions during cardiopulmonary resuscitation: improved outcome during a simulated single lay rescuer scenario. *Circulation* 2002;**105**:645–9.

205. Babbs CF, Nadkarni V. Optimizing chest compression to rescue ventilation ratios during one-rescuer CPR by professionals and lay persons: children are not just little adults. *Resuscitation* 2004;**61**:173–81.

206. Berg RA, Hilwig RW, Kern KB, Babar I, Ewy GA. Simulated mouth-to-mouth ventilation and chest compressions (bystander cardiopulmonary resuscitation) improves outcome in a swine model of prehospital pediatric asphyxia cardiac arrest. *Crit Care Med* 1999;**27**:1893–9.

207. Berg RA, Hilwig RW, Kern KB, et al. 'Bystander' chest compressions and assisted ventilation independently improve outcome from piglet asphyxia pulseless 'cardiac arrest'. *Circulation* 2000;**101**:1743–8.

208. Idris AH, Becker LB, Fuerst RS, et al. Effect of ventilation on resuscitation in an animal model of cardiac arrest. *Circulation* 1994;**90**:3063–9.

209. Babbs CF, Kern KB. Optimum compression to ventilation ratios in CPR under realistic, practical conditions: a physiological and mathematical analysis. *Resuscitation* 2002;**54**:147–57.

210. Hemway RJ, Christman C, Perlman J. The 3:1 is superior to a 15:2 ratio in a newborn manikin model in terms of quality of chest compressions and number of ventilations. *Arch Dis Child Fetal Neonatal Ed* 2013;**98**:F42–5.

211. Solevåg AL, Madland JM, Gjærum E, Nakstad B. Minute ventilation at different compression to ventilation ratios, different ventilation rates, and continuous chest compressions with asynchronous ventilation in a newborn manikin. *Scand J Trauma Resusc Emerg Med* 2012;**20**:73.

212. Solevåg AL, Dannevig I, Wyckoff M, et al. Extended series of cardiac compressions during CPR in a swine model of perinatal asphyxia. *Resuscitation* 2010;**81**:1571–6.

213. Solevåg AL, Dannevig I, Wyckoff M, Saugstad OD, Nakstad B. Return of spontaneous circulation with a compression:ventilation ratio of 15:2 versus 3:1 in newborn pigs with cardiac arrest due to asphyxia. *Arch Dis Child Fetal Neonatal Ed* 2011;**96**:F417–21.

214. Schmölzer GM, O'Reilly M, Labossiere J, et al. 3:1 compression to ventilation ratio versus continuous chest compression with asynchronous ventilation in a porcine model of neonatal resuscitation. *Resuscitation* 2014;**85**:270–5.

215. Sims DG, Heal CA, Bartle SM. The use of adrenaline and atropine in neonatal resuscitation. *Arch Dis Child Fetal Neonatal Ed* 1994;**70**: F3–10.

216. O'Donnell AI, Gray PH, Rogers YM. Mortality and neurodevelopmental outcome for infants receiving adrenaline in neonatal resuscitation. *J Paediatr Child Health* 1988;**34**:551–6.

217. Diamond LK, Allen FH Jr, Thomas WO Jr. Erythroblastosis fetalis. VII. Treatment with exchange transfusion. *N Engl J Med* 1951;**244**:39–49.

218. Hall RT, Rhodes PG. Total parenteral alimentation via indwelling umbilical catheters in the newborn period. *Arch Dis Child* 1976;**51**:929–34.

219. Linde LM, Higashino SM, Berman G, et al. Umbilical vessel cardiac catheterization and angiocardiography. *Circulation* 1966;**34**:984–8.

220. Prinz SC, Cunningham MD. Umbilical vessel catheterization. *J Fam Pract* 1980;**10**:885–90.

221. Ellemunter H, Simma B, Trawoger R, Maurer H. Intraosseous lines in preterm and full term neonates. *Arch Dis Child Fetal Neonatal Ed* 1999;**80**:F74–5.

222. Rajani AK, Chitkara R, Oehlert J, *et al*. Comparison of umbilical venous and intraosseous access during simulated neonatal resuscitation. *Pediatrics* 2011;**128**:e954–8.

223. Abe KK, Blum GT, Yamamoto LG. Intraosseous is faster and easier than umbilical venous catheterization in newborn emergency vascular access models. *Am J Emerg Med* 2000;**18**:126–9.

224. Costa S, De Carolis MP, Savarese I, *et al*. An unusual complication of umbilical catheterisation. *Eur J Pediatr* 2008;**167**:1467–9.

225. Lindemann R. Resuscitation of the newborn with endotracheal administration of epinephrine. *Acta Paed Scand* 1984;**73**:210–2.

226. Modest VE, Butterworth JF 4th. Effect of pH and lidocaine on betaadrenergic receptor binding: interaction during resuscitation. *Chest* 1995;**108**:1373–9.

227. Redding JS, Asuncion JS, Pearson JW. Effective routes of drug administration during cardiac arrest. *Anesth Analg (Clev)* 1967;**46**:253–8.

228. Redding JS, Pearson JW. Evaluation of drugs for cardiac resuscitation. *Anesthesiology* 1963;**24**:203–7.

229. Otto CW, Yakaitis RW, Blitt CD. Mechanism of action of epinephrine in resuscitation from asphyxial arrest. *Crit Care Med* 1981;**9**:321–4.

230. Michael JR, Guerci AD, Koehler RC, *et al*. Mechanisms by which epinephrine augments cerebral and myocardial perfusion during cardiopulmonary resuscitation in dogs. *Circulation* 1984;**69**:822–35.

231. Paradis NA, Martin GB, Rivers EP, *et al*. Coronary perfusion pressure and the return of spontaneous circulation in human cardiopulmonary resuscitation. *JAMA* 1990;**263**:1106–13.

232. Redding JS, Pearson JW. Resuscitation from ventricular fibrillation. *JAMA* 1968;**203**:255–60.

233. Brown CG, Werman HA, Davis EA, *et al*. The effects of graded doses of epinephrine on regional myocardial flow during cardiopulmonary resuscitation in swine. *Circulation* 1987;**75**:491–7.

234. Lindner KH, Ahnefeld FW, Bowdler IM. Comparison of different doses of epinephrine on myocardial perfusion and resuscitation success during cardiopulmonary resuscitation in a pig model. *Am J Emerg Med* 1991;**9**:27–31.

235. Perondi MB, Reis AG, Paiva EF, *et al*. A comparison of high-dose and standard-dose epinephrine in children with cardiac arrest. *N Engl J Med* 2004;**350**:1722–30.

236. Berg RA, Otto CW, Kern KB, *et al*. A randomized, blinded trial of high-dose epinephrine versus standard-dose epinephrine in a swine model of pediatric asphyxial cardiac arrest. *Crit Care Med* 1996;**24**:1695–700.

237. Pasternak JF, Groothuis DR, Fisher DP. Regional cerebral blood flow in the beagle puppy model of neonatal intraventricular hemorrhage: studies in systemic hypertension. *Neurology* 1983;**33**:559–66.

238. Basu P, Som S, Choudhuri N, *et al*. Contribution of the blood glucose level in perinatal asphyxia. *Eur J Pediatr* 2009;**168**:833–8.

239. Nadeem M, Murray DM, Boylan GB, *et al*. Early blood glucose profile and neurodevelopmental outcome at two years in neonatal hypoxic-ischaemic encephalopathy. *BMC Pediatr* 2011;**11**:10.

240. Salhab WA, Wyckoff MH, Laptook AR, *et al*. Initial hypoglycemia and neonatal brain injury in term infants with severe fetal acidemia. *Pediatrics* 2004;**114**:361–6.

241. Skellet S, Mayer A, Durward A, *et al*. Chasing the base deficit: hyperchloraemic acidosis following 0.9% saline fluid resuscitation. *Arch Dis Child* 2000;**83**:514–6.

242. O'Donnell CPF, Stenson BJ. Respiratory strategies for preterm infants. *Semin Fetal Neonatal Med* 2008;**13**:401–9.

243. Mercer JS, Vohr BR, McGrath MM, *et al*. Delayed cord clamping in very preterm infants reduces the incidence of intraventricular hemorrhage and late-onset sepsis - a randomized-controlled trial. *Pediatrics* 2006;**117**:1235–42.

244. Rabe H, Diaz-Rossello JL, Duley L, Dowswell T. Effect of timing of umbilical cord clamping and other strategies to influence placental transfusion at preterm birth on maternal and infant outcomes. *Cochrane Database Syst Rev* 2012;**8**: CD003248.

245. Backes CH, Rivera BK, Haque U, *et al*. Placental transfusion strategies in very preterm neonates: a systematic review and metaanalysis. *Obstet Gynecol* 2014;**124**:47–56.

246. Airey RJ, Farrar D, Duley L. Alternative positions for the baby at birth before clamping the umbilical cord. *Cochrane Database Syst Rev* 2010;**10**:CD007555.

247. Vain NE, Satragno DS, Gorenstein AN, *et al*. Effect of gravity on volume of placental transfusion: a multicentre, randomised, non-inferiority trial. *Lancet* 2014;**384**:235–40.

248. Al-Wassia H, Shah PS. Efficacy and safety of umbilical cord milking at birth: a systematic review and meta-analysis. *JAMA Pediatr* 2015;**169**:18–25.

249. Farrar D, Duley L, Burls A, *et al*. Rushing to clamp umbilical cord. More evidence is needed to inform practice. *Brit Med J* 2011;**342**:d122

250. Stanley FJ, Alberman ED. Infants of very low birthweight. 1. Factors affecting survival. *Dev Med Child Neurol* 1978;**20**:300–12.

251. Merritt TA, Farrell PM. Diminished pulmonary lecithin synthesis in acidosis: Experimental findings as related to the respiratory distress syndrome. *Pediatrics* 1976;**57**:32–40.

252. Knobel RB, Wimmer JE, Holbert D. Heat loss prevention for preterm infants in the delivery room. *J Perinatol* 2005;**25**:304–8.

253. McCall EM, Alderdice FA, Halliday HL, *et al*. Interventions to prevent hypothermia in preterm and/or low birthweight babies. *Cochrane Database Syst Rev* 2008;**1**:CD004210.

254. Vohra S, Roberts RS, Zhang B, *et al*. Heat Loss Prevention (HeLP) in the delivery room: A randomized controlled trial of polyethylene occlusive skin wrapping in very preterm infants. *J Pediatr* 2004;**145**:750–3.

255. Belsches TC, Tilly AE, Miller TR, *et al*. Randomized trial of plastic bags to prevent term neonatal hypothermia in a resource-poor setting. *Pediatrics* 2013;**132**:e656–61.

256. Leadford AE, Warren JB, Manasyan A, *et al*. Plastic bags for prevention of hypothermia in preterm and low birth weight infants. *Pediatrics* 2013;**132**:e128–34.

257. Bjorklund LJ, Ingimarsson J, Curstedt T, *et al*. Manual ventilation with a few large breaths at birth compromises the therapeutic effect of subsequent surfactant. *Pediatr Res* 1997;**42**:348–55.

258. Johnston ED, Stenson BJ. Am I getting chest wall movement? *Arch Dis Child Fetal Neonatal Ed* 2010;**95**:F391–2.

259. Morley CJ, Davis PG, Doyle L, *et al*. Nasal CPAP or intubation for very preterm infants. *New Engl J Med* 2008;**358**:700–8.

260. Ingimarsson J, Björklund LJ, Curstedt T. Incomplete protection by prophylactic surfactant against the adverse effects of large lung inflation in immature lambs at birth. *Intensive Care Med* 2004;**30**:1446–53.

261. Lundstrøm KE, Pryds O, Greisen G. Oxygen at birth and prolonged cerebral vasoconstriction in preterm infants. *Arch Dis Childhood Fetal Neonatal Ed* 1995;**73**:F81–6.

262. Vento M, Moro M, Escrig R, *et al*. Preterm resuscitation with low oxygen causes less oxidative stress, inflammation, and chronic lung disease. *Pediatrics* 2009;**124**:e439–49.

263. Rabi Y, Dawson JA. Oxygen therapy and oximetry in the delivery room. *Semin Fetal Neonatal Med* 2013;**18**:330–5.

264. American Thoracic Society / European Respiratory Society. Respiratory mechanics in infants: physiologic evaluation in health and disease. *Am Rev Respir Dis* 1993;**147**:474–96.

265. Schmölzer GM, Kamlin OC, O'Donnell CP, *et al*. Assessment of tidal volume and gas leak during mask ventilation of preterm infants in the delivery room. *Arch Dis Child Fetal Neonatal Ed* 2010;**95**:F393–7.

266. Poulton DA, Schmölzer GM, Morley CJ, Davis PG. Assessment of chest rise during mask ventilation of preterm infants in the delivery room. *Resuscitation* 2011;**82**:175–9.

267. Birch S, Rhodes H, Wylie P. Laryngeal damage from intubation (case report). *Br Med J* 1999;**318**:614.

268. Verder H, Albertsen P, Ebbesen F. *et al*. Nasal continuous positive airway pressure and early surfactant therapy for respiratory distress syndrome in newborns of less than 30 weeks gestation. *Pediatrics* 1999;**103**:e24.

269. Morley CJ. Systematic review of prophylactic vs rescue surfactant. *Arch Dis Child Fetal Neonatal Ed* 1997;**77**:F70–4.

270. Richmond S, Goldsmith JP. Refining the role of oxygen administration during delivery room resuscitation: What are the future goals? *Semin Fetal Neonatal Med* 2008;**13**:368–74.

271. Tan A, Schulze A, O'Donnell CP, Davis PG. Air versus oxygen for resuscitation of infants at birth. *Cochrane Database Syst Rev* 2005;**2**:CD002273.

272. National Institute for Health and Care Excellence (NICE). Intrapartum care: care of healthy women and their babies during childbirth. Clinical Guideline 190 (CG190). National Institute for Health and Care Excellence. London, 2014. (www.nice.org.uk/guidance/cg190/resources/guidance-intrapartum-care-care-of-healthy-women-and-their-babies-during-childbirth-pdf)

273. Hadar A, Rabinovich A, Sheiner E, *et al*. Obstetric characteristics and neonatal outcome of unplanned out-of-hospital term deliveries: a prospective, case-control study. *J Reprod Med* 2005;**50**:832–6.

274. Department of Health. The National Service Framework for Children and Young People. Maternity Services. Standard 11. London: Department of Health; 2004

275. Welsh Assembly Children's Health and Social Care Directorate. National Service Framework for Children, Young People and Maternity Services in Wales. Cardiff: Welsh Assembly Government; 2005.

276. Scottish Executive. A Framework for Maternity Services in Scotland. Edinburgh: Scottish Executive; 2001

277. Royal College of Midwives. Home Birth Hand Book: Volume 1: Promoting Home Birth. London: RCM; 2002.

278. Royal College of Midwives. Home Birth Hand Book: Volume 2: Practising Home Birth. London: RCM; 2003.

279. Brocklehurst P, Hardy P, Hollowell J, et al; Birthplace in England Collaborative Group. Perinatal and maternal outcomes by planned place of birth for healthy women with low risk pregnancies: the Birthplace in England national prospective cohort study. Brit Med J 2011;**343**:d7400.

280. McLelland GE, Morgans AE, McKenna LG. Involvement of emergency medical services at unplanned births before arrival to hospital: a structured review. Emerg Med J 2014;**31**:345–50.

281. Okumura A, Hayakawa F, Kato T, et al. Hypocarbia in preterm infants with periventricular leukomalacia: the relation between hypocarbia and mechanical ventilation. Pediatrics 2001;**107**:469–75.

282. Sweet DG, Carnielli V, Greisen G, et al. European consensus guidelines on the management of neonatal respiratory distress syndrome in preterm infants—2013 update. Neonatology 2013;**103**:353–68.

283. Akinloye O, O'Connell C, Allen AC, El-Naggar W. Post-resuscitation care for neonates receiving positive pressure ventilation at birth. Pediatrics 2014;**134**:e1057–62.

284. British Association of Perinatal Medicine. Newborn Early Warning Trigger and Track (NEWTT): A Framework for Practice. BAPM, 2015.

285. Holme H, Bhatt R, Koumettou M, Griffin MA, Winckworth LC. Retrospective evaluation of a new neonatal trigger score. Pediatrics 2013;**131**:e837–42.

286. Roland D, Madar J, Connolly G. The Newborn Early Warning (NEW) system: development of an at-risk infant intervention system. Infant 2010;**6**:116–20.

287. Cabal LA, Devaskar U, Siassi B, et al. Cardiogenic shock associated with perinatal asphyxia in preterm infants. J Pediatr 1980;**96**:705–10.

288. Thiebault DW, Hall FK, Sheehan MB, Hall RT. Postasphyxial lung disease in newborn infants with severe perinatal acidosis. Am J Obstet Gynecol 1984;**150**:393–9.

289. Robertson CMT, Finer NN, Grace MGA. School performance in survivors of neonatal encephalopathy associated with birth asphyxia at term. J Pediatr 1989;**114**:753–60.

290. Armstrong L, Stenson B. The effect of delayed sampling on umbilical cord arterial and venous lactate and blood gases in clamped and unclamped vessels. Arch Dis Child Fetal Neonatal Ed 2006;**91**:F342–5.

291. Goldenberg RL, Huddleston JF, Nelson KG. Apgar scores and umbilical arterial pH in preterm infants. Am J Obstet Gynecol 1984;**149**:651–4.

292. Johnson JWC, Richards DS, Wagaman RA. The case for routine umbilical blood acid-base studies at delivery. Am J Obstet Gynecol 1990;**162**:621–5.

293. Westgate J, Garibaldi JM, Greene KR. Umbilical cord blood gas analysis at delivery: a time for quality data. Br J Obstet Gynaecol 1994;**101**:1054–63.

294. Wong L, MacLennan AH. Gathering the evidence: cord gases and placental histology for births with low Apgar scores. Aust N Z J Obstet Gynaecol 2011;**51**:17–21.

295. Pelikan DM, Scherjon SA, Kanhai HH. The incidence of large fetomaternal hemorrhage and the Kleihauer-Betke test. Obstet Gynecol 2005;**106**:642–3.

296. Patient Safety Alert. Resources to support the prompt recognition of sepsis and the rapid initiation of treatment. Alert reference number: NHS/PSA/R/2014/015. NHS England, September 2014.

297. Leahy FAN, Cates D, MacCallum M, Rigatto H. Effect of CO_2 and 100% O_2 on cerebral blood flow in preterm infants. J Appl Physiol 1980;**48**:468–72.

298. Klinger G, Beyene J, Shah P, Perlman M. Do hyperoxaemia and hypercapnia add to the risk of brain injury after intrapartum asphyxia? Arch Dis Child Fetal Neonatal Ed 2005;**90**:49–52.

299. Kluckow M, Evans N. Low systemic blood flow in the preterm infant. Semin Neonatol 2001;**6**:75–84.

300. Ainsworth SB. Neonatal Formulary: Drug Use in Pregnancy and the First Year of Life. 7th edition. BMJ books. Wiley-Blackwell, Oxford, 2014. pp. 44–47.

301. Finer NN, Robertson CM, Richards RT, et al. Hypoxic-ischemic encephalopathy in term neonates: perinatal factors and outcome. J Pediatr 1981;**98**:112–7.

302. Kurinczuk JJ, White-Koning M, Badawi N. Epidemiology of neonatal encephalopathy and hypoxic-ischaemic encephalopathy. Early Hum Dev 2010;**86**:329–38.

303. Department of Health. An organisation with a memory. Report of an expert group on learning from adverse events in the NHS, chaired by the Chief Medical Officer. London: The Stationery Office; 2000.

304. National Institute for Health and Care Excellence (NICE). Therapeutic hypothermia with intracorporeal temperature monitoring for hypoxic perinatal brain injury: guidance. NICE interventional procedure guidance [IPG347]. London, 2010. (www.nice.org.uk/nicemedia/live/11315/48809/48809.pdf)

305. BAPM. Position statement on Therapeutic Cooling for Neonatal Encephalopathy. British Association of Perinatal Medicine 2010.

306. Kendall GS, Kapetanakis A, Ratnavel N, et al. Passive cooling for initiation of therapeutic hypothermia in neonatal encephalopathy. Arch Dis Child Fetal Neonatal Ed 2010;**95**:F408–12.

307. Levene M. Cool treatment for asphyxia, but what's next? Arch Dis Child Fetal Neonatal Ed 2010;**95**:F154–7.

308. Yamada NK, Halamek LP. On the need for precise, concise communication during resuscitation: a proposed solution. J Pediatr 2015;**166**:184–7.

309. Editorial. Anoxia in the newborn. Lancet 1951;**ii**:821–2.

310. NMC. Record keeping: Guidance for nurses and midwives. Nursing & Midwifery Council, London 2010.

311. Shankaran S (ed). Perinatal asphyxia. Clin Perinatol 1993;**20**:287–505.

312. Morland TA, Brice JEM, Walker CHM, Parija AC. Naloxone pharmacokinetics in the newborn. Br J Clin Pharmacol 1979;**9**:609–12.

313. Kasdorf E, Engel M, Heier L, Perlman JM. Therapeutic hypothermia in neonates and selective hippocampal injury on diffusion-weighted magnetic resonance imaging. Pediatr Neurol 2014;**51**:104–8.

314. Laptook AR, Shankaran S, Ambalavanan N, et al; Hypothermia Subcommittee of the NICHD Neonatal Research Network. Outcome of term infants using apgar scores at 10 minutes following hypoxic-ischemic encephalopathy. Pediatrics 2009;**124**:1619–26.

315. Sarkar S, Bhagat I, Bapuraj JR, et al. Does clinical status 1 week after therapeutic hypothermia predict brain MRI abnormalities? J Perinatol 2013;**33**:538–42.

316. Nuffield Council on Bioethics. Critical care decisions in fetal and neonatal medicine: ethical issues. Nuffield Council on Bioethics, 2006.

317. Wilkinson AR, Ahluwalia J, Cole A, et al. Management of babies born extremely preterm at less than 26 weeks of gestation: a framework for clinical practice at the time of birth. Arch Dis Child Fetal Neonatal Ed 2009;**94**:F2–5.

318. Tin W, Wariyar U, Hey E. Changing prognosis for babies of less than 28 weeks gestation in the north of England between 1983 and 1994. Br Med J 1997;**314**:107–11.

319. Wood NS, Marlow N, Costeloe K, et al. Neurologic and developmental disability after extremely preterm birth. N Engl J Med 2000;**343**:374–84.

320. Costeloe KL, Hennessy EM, Haider S, et al. Short term outcomes after extreme preterm birth in England: comparison of two birth cohorts in 1995 and 2006 (the EPICure studies). Brit Med J 2012;**345**:e7976.

321. Macfarlane PI, Wood S, Bennett J. Non-viable delivery at 20-23 weeks gestation: observations and signs of life after birth. Arch Dis Child Fetal Neonatal Ed 2003;**88**:F199–202.

322. Royal College of Paediatrics and Child Health. Withholding or withdrawing life sustaining treatment in children—a framework for practice. 2nd edn. London: RCPCH, 2004.

323. Riesenberg LA, Leitzsch J, Little BW. Systematic review of handoff mnemonics literature. Am J Med Qual 2009;**24**:196–204.

324. Marini V, (ed). The SBAR technique: improves communication, enhances patient safety. Jt Comm Perspect Patient Saf 2005;**5**:1–2,8.

325. Vergales BD, Dwyer EJ, Wilson SM, et al. NASCAR pit-stop model improves delivery room and admission efficiency and outcomes for infants <27 weeks' gestation. Resuscitation 2015;**92**:7–13.

326. Thomas EJ, Sexton JB, Lasky RE, et al. Teamwork and quality during neonatal care in the delivery room. J Perinatol 2006;**26**:163–9.

327. Greig PR, Higham H, Nobre AC. Failure to perceive clinical events: An under-recognised source of error. Resuscitation 2014;**85**:952–6.

328. Norris EM, Lockey AS. Human factors in resuscitation teaching. Resuscitation 2012;**83**:423 –7.

329. Andersen PO, Jensen MK, Lippert A, et al. Identifying non-technical skills and barriers for improvement of teamwork in cardiac arrest teams. Resuscitation 2010;**81**:695–702.

330. Høyer CB, Christensen EF, Eika B. Junior physician skill and behaviour in resuscitation: a simulation study. *Resuscitation* 2009;**2**:244–8.

331. Goleman D. Leadership that gets results. *Harvard Business Review* 2000;March–April:79–90.

332. Reason J. The contribution of latent human failures to the breakdown of complex systems. *Phil Trans R Soc Lond* 1990;**327**:475–84.

333. Reason J. Combating omission errors through task analysis and good reminders. *Qual Saf Health Care* 2002;**11**:40–4.

334. Thomas EJ, Taggart B, Crandell S, et al. Teaching teamwork during the Neonatal Resuscitation Program: a randomized trial. *J Perinatol* 2007;**27**:409–14.

335. Thomas EJ, Williams AL, Reichman EF, et al. Team training in the neonatal resuscitation program for interns: teamwork and quality of resuscitations. *Pediatrics* 2010;**125**:539–46.

336. Williams AL, Lasky RE, Dannemiller JL, et al. Teamwork behaviours and errors during neonatal resuscitation. *Qual Saf Health Care* 2010;**19**:60–4.

337. Mosley CM, Shaw BN. A longitudinal cohort study to investigate the retention of knowledge and skills following attendance on the Newborn Life support course. *Arch Dis Child* 2013;**98**:582–6.

338. Kohn LT, Corrigan JM, Donaldson MS eds. *To Err is Human. Building a Safer Health System*. Washington, DC: National Academy Press, 1999. (full text available on-line at www.nap.edu/books/0309068371/html)

339. Couper K, Perkins GD. Debriefing after resuscitation. *Curr Opin Crit Care* 2013;**19**:188–94.

340. Kane K, Swearingen C, Dyamenahalli U. Critical incident debriefing after cardiopulmonary resuscitation in pediatric cardiac ICU: Effect on patient safety, performance improvement and survey. *Circulation* 2012;**126** (suppl 1):A252.

341. Allbutt C. Diseases of the arteries including angina pectoris, vol 1. London: Macmillan, 1915, p 154.

342. Daga SR, Dave K, Mehta V, Pai V. Tracheal suction in meconium stained infants: a randomized controlled study. *J Trop Pediatr* 1994;**40**:198–200.

343. Linder N, Aranda JV, Tsur M, et al. Need for endotracheal intubation and suction in meconium-stained neonates. *J Pediatr* 1988;**112**:613–5.

344. Liu WF, Harrington T. The need for delivery room intubation of thin meconium in the low-risk newborn: a clinical trial. *Am J Perinatol* 1998;**15**:675–82.

345. Ersdal HL, Mduma E, Svensen E, Perlman JM. Early initiation of basic resuscitation interventions including face mask ventilation may reduce birth asphyxia related mortality in low-income countries: a prospective descriptive observational study. *Resuscitation* 2012;**83**:869–73.

346. Brady JP, James LS, Baker MA. Heart rate changes in the fetus and newborn infant during labor, delivery and the immediate neonatal period. *Am J Obstet Gynecol* 1962;**84**:1–12.

347. Peltonen T. Placental transfusion - advantage and disadvantage. *Eur J Pediatr* 1981;**137**:141–6 .

348. Yao AC, Hirvensalo M, Lind J. Placental transfusion-rate and uterine contraction. *Lancet* 1968;**i**:380–3.

349. Vanhaesebrouck P, Vanneste K, de Praeter C, et al. Tight nuchal cord and neonatal hypovolaemic shock. *Arch Dis Child* 1987;**62**:1276–7.

350. Mercer J, Erickson-Owens D, Skovgaard R. Cardiac asystole at birth: is hypovolemic shock the cause? *Med Hypotheses* 2009;**72**:458–63.

351. Baenziger O, Stolkin F, Keel M, et al. The influence of the timing of cord clamping on postnatal cerebral oxygenation in preterm neonates: a randomized, controlled trial. *Pediatrics* 2007;**119**:455–9.

352. Tolosa JN, Dong-Hyuk P, Eve DJ, et al. Mankind's first natural stem cell transplant. *J Cell Mol Med* 2010;**14**:488–95.

353. Dunn PM. Postnatal placental respiration. *Dev Med Child Neurol* 1966;**8**:607–8.

354. World Health Organisation. WHO recommendations for the prevention and treatment of postpartum haemorrhage. World Health Organization, Geneva, Switzerland, 2012

355. RCOG Scientific Advisory Committee. Clamping of the umbilical cord and placental transfusion. Royal College of Obstetricians and Gynaecologists Opinion Paper 14, 2009.

356. Perlman JM, Wyllie J, Kattwinkel J, et al. Part 11: neonatal resuscitation: 2010 International consensus on cardiopulmonary resuscitation and emergency cardiovascular care science with treatment recommendations. *Circulation* 2010;**122** (suppl 2):S516–38.

357. Wyllie J, Perlman J, Kattwinkel J, et al. 2010 International consensus on cardiopulmonary resuscitation and emergency cardiovascular care science with treatment recommendations: Neonatal resuscitation. *Resuscitation* 2010;**81S**:e260–87.

358. Erickson-Owens DA, Mercer JS, Oh W. Umbilical cord milking in term infants delivered by cesarean section: a randomized controlled trial. *J Perinatol* 2012;**32**:580–4.

359. Walsh SZ. Early clamping versus stripping of cord: comparative study of electrocardiogram in neonatal period. *Br Heart J* 1969;**31**:122–6.

360. Takami T, Suganami Y, Sunohara D, et al. Umbilical cord milking stabilizes cerebral oxygenation and perfusion in infants born before 29 weeks of gestation. *J Pediatr* 2012;**161**:742–7.

361. Hosono S, Mugishima H, Fujita H, et al. Blood pressure and urine output during the first 120 h of life in infants born at less than 29 weeks' gestation related to umbilical cord milking. *Arch Dis Child Fetal Neonatal Ed* 2009;**94**:F328–31.

362. Upadhyay A, Gothwal S, Parihar R, et al. Effect of umbilical cord milking in term and near term infants: randomized control trial. *Am J Obstet Gynecol* 2013;**208**:e121–6.

363. Walsh SZ. Early versus late clamping of the cord: a comparative study of the ECG in the neonatal period. *Biol Neonat* 1968;**12**:343–57.

364. Rabe H, Jewison A, Alvarez RF, et al. Milking compared with delayed cord clamping to increase placental transfusion in preterm neonates: a randomized controlled trial. *Obstet Gynecol* 2011;**117**:205–11.

365. Katheria AC, Leone TA, Woelkers D, et al. The effects of umbilical cord milking on hemodynamics and neonatal outcomes in premature neonates. *J Pediatr* 2014;**164**:1045–50.e1.

366. Jobe AH, Kramer BW, Moss TJ, et al. Decreased indicators of lung injury with continuous positive expiratory pressure in preterm lambs. *Pediatr Res* 2002;**52**:387–92.

367. Probyn ME, Hooper SB, Dargaville PA, et al. Positive end expiratory pressure during resuscitation of premature lambs rapidly improves blood gases without adversely affecting arterial pressure. *Pediatr Res* 2004;**56**:198–204.

368. Finer NN, Carlo WA, Walsh MC, et al. Early CPAP versus surfactant in extremely preterm infants. *N Engl J Med* 2010;**362**:1970–9.

369. Dunn MS, Kaempf J, de Klerk A, et al. Randomized trial comparing 3 approaches to the initial respiratory management of preterm neonates. *Pediatrics* 2011;**128**:e1069–76.

370. Rojas-Reyes MX, Morley CJ, Soll R. Prophylactic versus selective use of surfactant in preventing morbidity and mortality in preterm infants. *Cochrane Database Syst Rev* 2012;**3**:CD000510.

371. Kosch PC, Hutchison AA, Wozniak JA, et al. Posterior cricoarytenoid and diaphragm activities during tidal breathing in neonates. *J Appl Physiol* 1988;**64**:1968–78.

372. Kosch PC, Stark AR. Dynamic maintenance of end-expiratory lung-volume in full-term infants. *J Appl Physiol* 1984;**57**:1126–33.

373. Fox WW, Gutsche BB, DeVore JS. A delivery room approach to the meconium aspiration syndrome (MAS). Immediate intubation, endotracheal suction, and oxygen administration can reduce morbidity and mortality. *Clin Pediatr (Phila)* 1977;**16**:325–8.

374. Gregory GA, Gooding CA, Phibbs RH, et al. Meconium aspiration in infants—a prospective study. *J Pediatr* 1974;**85**:848–52.

375. Carson BS, Losey RW, Bowes WA Jr, Simmons MA. Combined obstetric and pediatric approach to prevent meconium aspiration syndrome. *Am J Obstet Gynecol* 1976;**126**:712–5.

376. Rossi EM, Philipson EH, Williams TG, et al. Meconium aspiration syndrome: Intrapartum and neonatal attributes. *Am J Obstet Gynecol* 1989;**161**:1106–10.

377. Wiswell TE, Tuggle JM, Turner BS. Meconium aspiration syndrome: have we made a difference? *Pediatrics* 1990; **85**:715–21.

378. Davis RO, Philips JB 3rd, Harris BA Jr, et al. Fatal meconium aspiration syndrome occurring despite airway management considered appropriate. *Am J Obstet Gynecol* 1985;**151**:731–6.

379. Halliday HL. Endotracheal intubation at birth for preventing morbidity and mortality in vigorous, meconium-stained infants born at term. *Cochrane Database Syst Rev* 2001;**1**:CD000500.

380. Bhat R, Vidyasagar D. Delivery room management of meconium-stained infant. *Clin Perinatol* 2012;**39**:817–31.

381. Hein HA. The use of sodium bicarbonate in neonatal resuscitation: help or harm. *Pediatrics* 1993;**91**:496–7.

382. Ascher JL, Poland RL. Sodium bicarbonate: basically useless therapy. *Pediatrics* 2008;**122**:831–5.

383. Sáenz P, Brugada M, de Jongh B, et al. A survey of intravenous sodium bicarbonate in neonatal asphyxia among European neonatologists: gaps between scientific evidence and clinical practice. *Neonatology* 2011;**99**:170–6.

384. Lokesh L, Kumar P, Murki S, et al. A randomized controlled trial of sodium bicarbonate in neonatal resuscitation: effect on immediate outcome. *Resuscitation* 2004;**60**:219–23

385. Murki S, Kumar P, Lingappa L, *et al*. Effect of a single dose of sodium bicarbonate given during neonatal resuscitation at birth on the acid—base status on first day of life. *J Perinatol* 2004;**24**,696–9.

386. Preziosi MP, Roig JC, Hargrove N, *et al*. Metabolic acidemia with hypoxia attenuates the haemodynamic responses to epinephrine during resuscitation in lambs. *Crit Care Med* 1993;**21**:1901–7.

387. Raymondos K, Panning B, Leuwer M, *et al*. Absorption and hemodynamic effects of airway administration of adrenaline in patients with severe cardiac disease. *Ann Intern Med* 2000;**132**:800–3.

388. Kleinman ME, Oh W, Stonstreet BS. Comparison of intravenous and endotracheal epinephrine during cardiopulmonary resuscitation in newborn piglets. *Crit Care Med* 1999;**27**:2748–85.

389. Barber CA, Wyckoff MH. Use and efficacy of endotracheal versus intravenous epinephrine during neonatal cardiopulmonary resuscitation in the delivery room. *Pediatrics* 2006;**118**:1028–34.

390. Crespo SG, Schoffstall JM, Fuhs LR, Spivey WH. Comparison of two doses of endotracheal epinephrine in a cardiac arrest model. *Ann Emerg Med* 1991;**20**:230–4.

391. Jasani MS, Nadkarni VM, Finkelstein MS, *et al*. Effects of different techniques of endotracheal epinephrine administration in pediatric porcine hypoxic-hypercarbic cardiopulmonary arrest. *Crit Care Med* 1994;**22**:1174–80.

392. Gibbs J, Newson T, Williams J, Davidson DC. Naloxone hazard in infant of opioid abuser. *Lancet* 1989;**ii**:159–60.

393. Gupta N, Corbett H, Ismail R, *et al*. Allantoic cyst - an unusual umbilical cord swelling. *J Surg Case Rep* 2011;**2011**:5.

394. Mattei P. Urachal remnant perforation during umbilical vein catheterization in a newborn. *J Pediatr Surg* 2007;**42**:722–4.

395. Robinson JN, Abuhamad AZ. Abdominal wall and umbilical cord anomalies. *Clin Perinatol* 2000;**27**:947–78.

396. Karlberg P, Cherry RB, Escardo FE, *et al*. Pulmonary ventilation and mechanics of breathing in the first minutes of life, including the onset of respiration. *Acta Paediatr* 1962;**51**:121–36.

397. Harling AE, Beresford MW, Vince GS, *et al*. Does sustained lung inflation at resuscitation reduce lung injury in the preterm infant? *Arch Dis Child Fetal Neonatal Ed* 2005;**90**:F406–10.

398. Lindner W, Högel J, Pohlandt F. Sustained pressure-controlled inflation or intermittent mandatory ventilation in preterm infants in the delivery room? A randomized, controlled trial on initial respiratory support via nasopharyngeal tube. *Acta Paediatr* 2005;**94**:303–9.

399. Lista G, Boni L, Scopesi F, *et al*; SLI Trial Investigators. Sustained lung inflation at birth for preterm infants: a randomized clinical trial. *Pediatrics* 2015;**135**:e457–64.

400. Schmölzer GM, Kumar M, Aziz K, *et al*. Sustained inflation versus positive pressure ventilation at birth: a systematic review and meta-analysis. *Arch Dis Child Fetal Neonatal Ed* 2015;**100**:F361–8.

401. Yeomans ER, Hauth JC, Gilstrap LC 3rd, *et al*. Umbilical cord pH, PCO_2, and bicarbonate following uncomplicated term vaginal deliveries. *Am J Obstet Gynecol* 1985;**151**:798–800.

402. Fee SC, Malee K, Deddish R, *et al*. Severe acidosis and subsequent neurologic status. *Am J Obstet Gynecol* 1990;**162**:802–6.

403. Gilstrap LC 3rd, Leveno KJ, Burris J, *et al*. Diagnosis of birth asphyxia on the basis of fetal pH, Apgar score, and newborn cerebral dysfunction. *Am J Obstet Gynecol* 1989;**161**:825–30.

404. James LS, Weisbrot IM, Prince CE, *et al*. The acid base status of human infants in relation to birth asphyxia and the onset of respiration. *J Pediatr* 1958;**52**:379–94.

405. Goodwin TM, Belai I, Hernandez P, *et al*. Asphyxial complications in the term newborn with severe umbilical acidemia. *Am J Obstet Gynecol* 1992;**167**:1506–12.

406. Martin GC, Green RS, Holzman IR. Acidosis in newborns with nuchal cords and normal Apgar scores. *J Perinatol* 2005;**25**:162–5.

407. Johnson JW, Richards DS. The etiology of fetal acidosis as determined by umbilical cord acid-base studies. *Am J Obstet Gynecol* 1997;**177**:274–80.

408. Pomerance J. Umbilical cord blood gases casebook. Interpreting umbilical cord blood gases, VII. *J Perinatol* 2000;**20**:338–9.

409. Apgar V, James LS. Further observations on the Newborn Scoring System. *Am J Dis Child* 1962;**104**:419–28.

410. Lie KK, Groholt EK, Eskild A. Association of cerebral palsy with Apgar score in low and normal birthweight infants – a population based cohort study. *Br Med J* 2010;**341**:c4990.

411. Nelson KB, Ellenberg JH. Apgar scores as predictors of chronic neurological disability. *Pediatrics* 1981;**68**:36–44.

412. Stevens SS. On the theory of scales of measurement. *Science* 1946;**103**:677–80.

413. Sykes G, Molloy P, Johnson P, *et al*. Do Apgar scores indicate asphyxia? *Lancet* 1982;**i**:494–6.

414. Sarnat HB, Sarnat MS. Neonatal encephalopathy following fetal distress: a clinical and electroencephalographic study. *Arch Neurol* 1976;**33**:696–705.

415. Levene MI, Sands C, Grindelus H, Moore JR. Comparison of two methods of predicting outcome in perinatal asphyxia. *Lancet* 1986;**i**:67–9.

416. Abel F, Bajaj Y, Wyatt M, Wallis C. The successful use of the nasopharyngeal airway in Pierre Robin sequence: an 11-year experience. *Arch Dis Child* 2012;**97**:331–4.

417. Parhizkar N, Saltzman B, Grote K, *et al*. Nasopharyngeal airway for management of airway obstruction in infants with micrognathia. *Cleft Palate Craniofac J* 2011;**48**:478–82.

418. Roberts K, Whalley H, Bleetman A. The Nasopharyngeal airway: Dispelling myths and establishing the facts. *Emerg Med J* 2005;**22**:394–6.

419. Shen CM, Soong WJ, Jeng MJ, *et al*. Nasopharyngeal tract length measurement in infants. *Acta Paediatr Taiwan* 2002;**43**:82–5.

420. Heaf DP, Helms PJ, Dinwiddie R, *et al*. Nasopharyngeal airways in Pierre Robin Syndrome. *J Pediatr* 1982;**100**:698–703.

421. Roberts K, Porter K. How do you size a nasopharyngeal airway? *Resuscitation* 2003;**56**:19–23.

422. Gandini D, Brimacombe J. Manikin training for neonatal resuscitation with the laryngeal mask airway. *Paediatr Anaesth* 2004;**14**:493–4.

423. Galderisi A, De Bernardo G, Lorenzon E, Trevisanuto D. i-gel: a new supraglottic device for effective resuscitation of a very low birthweight infant with Cornelia de Lange syndrome. *BMJ Case Rep* 2015 Mar 25;2015.

424. McEvoy C, Sardesai S, Macri C, Paul R, Durand M. Neonatal pulmonary mechanics and oxygenation after prophylactic amnioinfusion in labor: a randomized clinical trial. *Pediatrics* 1995;**95**:688–92.

425. Barrie H. Resuscitation of the newborn. *Lancet* 1963;**i**:650–5.

426. Benfield DG, Flaksman RJ, Lin T-H, *et al*. Teaching intubation skills using newly deceased infants *JAMA* 1991;**265**:2360–3.

427. Orlowski JP, Kanoti GA, Mehlman MJ. The ethics of using newly dead patients for teaching and practicing intubation techniques. *New Engl J Med* 1988;**319**:439–41.

428. O'Donnell CP, Kamlin CO, Davis PG, Morley CJ. Endotracheal intubation attempts during neonatal resuscitation: success rates, duration and adverse effects. *Pediatrics* 2006;**117**:e16–21.

429. Kempley ST, Moreiras JW, Petrone FL. Endotracheal tube length for neonatal intubation. *Resuscitation* 2008;**77**:369–73.

430. Loew A, Thibeault DW. A new and safe method to control the depth of endotracheal intubation in neonates. *Pediatrics* 1974;**54**:506–8.

431. Gill I, O'Donnell CP. Vocal cord guides on neonatal endotracheal tubes. *Arch Dis Child Fetal Neonatal Ed* 2014;**99**:F344.

432. Yam CH, Dawson JA, Schmölzer GM, *et al*. Heart rate changes during resuscitation of newly born infants. *Arch Dis Child Fetal Neonatal Ed* 2011;**96**:F102–7.

433. Kamlin COF, O'Donnell CPF, Davis PG, *et al*. Colorimetric end-tidal carbon dioxide detectors in the delivery room: strengths and limitations. A case report. *J Pediatr* 2005;**147**:547–8.

434. Doss A. Resuscitation of the newborn. *Br Med J* 1964;**2**:1331–41.

435. Hosono S, Inami I, Fujita H, *et al*. A role of end-tidal CO_2 monitoring for assessment of tracheal intubations in very low birth weight infants during neonatal resuscitation at birth. *J Perinat Med* 2009;**37**:79–84.

436. Repetto JE, Donohue PK, Baker SF, *et al*. Use of capnography in the delivery room for assessment of endotracheal tube placement. *J Perinatol* 2001;**21**:284–7.

437. Roberts WA, Maniscalco WM, Cohen AR, *et al*. The use of capnography for recognition of esophageal intubation in the neonatal intensive care unit. *Pediatr Pulmonol* 1995;**19**:262–8.

438. Garey DM, Rich W, Heldt G, *et al*. Tidal volume threshold for colorimetric carbon dioxide detectors available for use in neonates. *Pediatrics* 2008;**121**:e1524–7.

439. Aziz HF, Martin JB, Moore JJ. The pediatric disposable end-tidal carbon dioxide detector role in endotracheal intubation in newborns. *J Perinatol* 1999;**19**:110–3.

440. Hughes SM, Blake BL, Woods SL, Lehmann CU. False-positive results on colorimetric carbon dioxide analysis in neonatal resuscitation: potential for serious patient harm. *J Perinatol* 2007;**27**:800–1.

441. Brattebø G, Wisborg T, Solheim K, Oyen N. Public opinion on different approaches to teaching intubation techniques. *Br Med J* 1993;**307**:1256–7.

NLS

442. Heinild S, Søndergaard T, Tudvad F. Bone marrow infusions in childhood: experiences from a thousand infusions. *J Pediatr* 1947;**30**:400–11.

443. Bohn D. Intraosseous vascular access: from the archives to the ABC. *Crit Care Med* 1999;**27**:1053–4.

444. Vidal R, Kissoon N, Gayle M. Compartment syndrome following intraosseous infusion. *Pediatrics* 1993;**91**:1201–2.

445. Oesterlie GE, Petersen KK, Knudsen L, *et al*. Crural amputation of a newborn as a consequence of intraosseous needle insertion and calcium infusion. *Pediatr Emerg Care* 2014;**30**:413–4.

446. La Flece FR, Slepin MJ, Vargasa J, *et al*. Iatrogenic bilateral tibial fractures after intraosseus infusion attempts in a 3-month-old infant. *Ann Emerg Med* 1989;**18**:1099–101.

447. Chawla S, Amaram A, Gopal SP, Natarajan G. Safety and efficacy of Trans-warmer mattress for preterm neonates: results of a randomized controlled trial. *J Perinatol* 2011;**31**:780–4.

448. Almeida PG, Chandley J, Davis J, Harrigan RC. Use of the heated gel mattress and its impact on admission temperature of very low birth-weight infants. *Adv Neonatal Care* 2009;**9**:34–9.

449. Thomas MR, Yoxall CW, Weeks AD, Duley L. Providing newborn resuscitation at the mother's bedside: assessing the safety, usability and acceptability of a mobile trolley. *BMC Pediatr* 2014;**14**:135.

450. Kaufman J, Schmölzer GM, Kamlin CO, *et al*. Mask ventilation of preterm infants in the delivery room. *Arch Dis Child Fetal Neonatal Ed* 2013;**98**:F405–10.

451. van Vonderen JJ, Kleijn TA, Schilleman K, *et al*. Compressive force applied to a manikin's head during mask ventilation. *Arch Dis Child Fetal Neonatal Ed* 2012;**97**:F254–8.

452. Hawkes CP, Oni OA, Dempsey EM, *et al*. Potential hazard of the Neopuff T piece resuscitator in the absence of flow limitation. *Arch Dis Child Fetal Neonatal Ed* 2009;**94**:F461–3.

453. Schilleman K, Schmölzer GM, Kamlin OC, *et al*. Changing gas flow during neonatal resuscitation: a manikin study. *Resuscitation* 2011;**82**:920–4.

454. Thakur A, Saluja S, Modi M, *et al*. T piece or self inflating bag for positive pressure ventilation during delivery room resuscitation: An RCT. *Resuscitation* 2015;**90**:21–4.

455. Hawkes CP, Ryan CA, Dempsey EM. Comparison of the T piece resuscitator with other neonatal manual ventilation devices: a qualitative review. *Resuscitation* 2012;**83**:797–802.

456. Thio M, Dawson JA, Moss TJ, *et al*. Self-inflating bags versus T piece resuscitator to deliver sustained inflations in a preterm lamb model. *Arch Dis Child Fetal Neonatal Ed* 2014;**99**:F274–7.

457. McHale S, Thomas M, Hayden E, *et al*. Variation in inspiratory time and tidal volume with T piece neonatal resuscitator: association with operator experience and distraction. *Resuscitation* 2008;79:230–3

458. Klingenberg C, Wheeler KI, Davis PG, *et al*. A practical guide to neonatal volume guarantee ventilation. *J Perinatol* 2011;**31**:575–85.

459. Schmolzer GM, Poulton DA, Dawson JA, *et al*. Assessment of flow waves and colorimetric CO_2 detector for endotracheal tube placement during neonatal resuscitation. *Resuscitation* 2011;**82**:307–12.

460. Mian QN, Pichler G, Binder C, *et al*. Tidal volumes in spontaneously breathing preterm infants supported with continuous positive airway pressure. *J Pediatr* 2014;**165**:702–6.e1.

461. Field D, Milner AD, Hopkin IE. Efficiency of manual resuscitators at birth. *Arch Dis Child* 1986;**61**:300–2.

462. Ainsworth SB, Humphreys R, Stewart L. The pressure is on! The danger of a broken blow off valve on a bag valve mask. *Arch Dis Child Fetal Neonatal Ed* 2006;**91**:F233.

463. Cushing P. Mis-assembly of adult and paediatric manual resuscitators. *Resuscitation* 2002;**55**:347–8.

464. O'Donnell CPF, Kamlin COF, Davis PG, Morley CJ. Obtaining pulse oximetry data in neonates: a randomised crossover study of sensor application techniques. *Arch Dis Child Fetal Neonatal Ed* 2005;**90**:F84–5.

465. Voogdt KG, Morrison AC, Wood FE, *et al*. A randomised, simulated study assessing auscultation of heart rate at birth. *Resuscitation* 2010;**81**:1000–3.

466. Kamlin CO, O'Donnell CP, Everest NJ, *et al*. Accuracy of clinical assessment of infant heart rate in the delivery room. *Resuscitation* 2006;**71**:319–21.

467. Adzick NS. Management of fetal lung lesions. *Clin Perinatol* 2009;**36**:363–76.

468. Scott RJ, Goodburn SF. Potter's syndrome in the second trimester—prenatal screening and pathological findings in 60 cases of oligohydramnios sequence. *Prenat Diagn* 1995;**15**:519–25.

NOTES

NEWBORN LIFE SUPPORT